THE
PROFESSIONAL
MEDICAL
INTERPRETER

A Comprehensive 40-Hour
Medical Interpreting Course

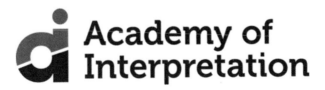
Academy of Interpretation

SECOND EDITION

Academy of Interpretation
1600 Spring Hill Road, Suite 210
Vienna, VA 22102
1-800-968-2919

WWW.ACADEMYOFINTERPRETATION.COM

Acknowledgements

We want to thank our families, friends and colleagues who are not mentioned for their great support and advice during the writing of this course.

This course was a labor of love for the founders and staff of the Academy of Interpretation. Plans for developing this course began in 2012. Our aspiration has been brought to life in a course developed based on accreditation standards and that gathered our experience and wisdom from being both an interpreting agency and interpreter training company. The largest effort to bring this course to completion spanned from late–2019 and throughout 2020–during the first year of the worldwide COVID-19 pandemic.

In addition to the writers, contributors, reviewers and staff mentioned below, we would also like to thank and acknowledge the healthcare providers, hospital language services managers and their staff who were kind enough to provide valuable feedback, and share their knowledge and experience that helped us in designing our medical interpreter course and accompanying textbook.

Special thanks to **Vanessa Niño** from MedStar Health for her mentorship and advice over the years.

We would like to acknowledge and express our gratitude to the following individuals who contributed to this course including the textbook, presentation materials, and implementation into a learning management system (LMS), so the course can be accessed online.

SAMEH ABDELKADER, Co-Founder and Director of Education for the Academy of Interpretation and Recipient of the 2015 IMIA Distinction in Education Award

For the direction, vision and contribution of his ten years' experience teaching adult learners the complex skills involved in becoming a professional medical interpreter.

Specifically, Mr. Abdelkader utilized our experiences in the Washington, D.C. metropolitan area, where the hospital systems expect the very best in terms of quality interpretation services. That combined with his wisdom and heart has allowed us to achieve success in training thousands of students both in-person, remotely by video conference, and through online training.

TIMOTHY WORSTER, Founder of Liberty Language Services

For the vision of developing and providing a world-class training that is affordable and accessible to all, with the ultimate goal of serving the communities where we live and work. Whether they be language access services staff within hospitals or individuals who meet the qualifications to be trained to give the gift of their language, culture, and voice to the limited-English-proficient (LEP) communities in the United States and beyond.

DREW BAHR, Esq., Spanish/English Legal and Medical Interpreter

Drew Bahr is a licensed immigration attorney, a medical and legal English/Spanish interpreter, and an interpreter trainer. Mr. Bahr was involved in the creation of the course content including presentation material.

CYNTHIA E. ROAT, MPH

Cindy Roat is an international consultant on language access in health care and patient navigation. A recognized subject matter expert on medical interpreting, she contributed the chapter and exercises on the topic of **message conversion:** the mechanics of converting a spoken message from one language into another.

IZABEL SOUZA, Ph.D.

Dr. Souza is an international expert and leader for medical interpreting. She served as reviewer and contributed to the book as a recognized subject matter expert in medical interpretation and intercultural mediation. Her chapter on The Roles of Interpreters emphasizes the undeniable cultural broker role and how medical interpreters mediate intercultural communication between patients and healthcare providers.

DR. JACQUELINE MESSING, Ph.D.

Dr. Messing is a linguistic anthropologist and served as reviewer and copy editor for the course textbook and presentation materials. Her research interests focus on issues of language, identity, ideology, race and racism in Mexico and the United States, on indigenous communities, multilingualism, and attempts to revitalize native languages through education. Dr. Messing's review was done in the context of the tumultuous year that was 2020 and she sought to also review for inclusivity, equality, and diversity.

···

MARIA BUENDIA, Certified Healthcare Interpreter for English/Spanish and Medical Interpreter Trainer

···

With a degree in microbiology and as an experienced healthcare interpreter, Ms. Schlenker is an in-house subject matter expert and provided her review of the course and contributed medical terminology content and exercises.

Additional Academy of Interpretation staff that contributed to the review, refinement, and editing include **Lia Cunanan** and **Devin Stewart**. Ms. Cunanan also coordinated beta testing of the online course.

Special recognition goes to **Salar Raoufi** who brought the course to life in its digital format, as well as providing project management. Mr. Raoufi contributed graphic content, interactivity to the online course, final touches, and LMS implementation to bring the course online and available to the world.

We would also like to acknowledge **medical interpreters** worldwide for their dedication to the field. Their commitment to working to serve their communities is admirable and serves as inspiration for the creation of all our trainings and especially this one. And a special acknowledgment to those interpreters who chose to continue to work in-person during the COVID-19 pandemic.

Table of Contents

Welcome

to the AOI's 40-Hour medical interpreter training course,
THE PROFESSIONAL MEDICAL INTERPRETER

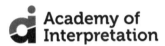

Welcome to the Academy of Interpretation. We are pleased to present this training to you as the next exciting step in your medical interpreting career. This course is for fully bilingual individuals who wish to start working as interpreters. This course is also catered to dedicated interpreters who may (1) not have previously been trained, (2) wish to refresh their knowledge and skills, and/or (3) want to build on their foundation of proper interpreting techniques and abilities, in a fun, collaborative setting.

Please note that the information in this welcome and introduction will not be tested. Also, the numbering of the sections in the textbook will skip some numbers to align with the course presentation.

> Accompanying Medical Terminology Textbook: Medical Terminology for Medical Interpreters, by the Academy of Interpretation, is the accompanying textbook to this comprehensive course.

THE IMIA AND NCIHC

The International Medical Interpreters Association (IMIA) and the National Council on Interpreting in Health Care (NCIHC) are the most important organizations for medical and healthcare interpreting in the U.S. Both organizations have developed standards of practice and code of ethics that are necessary parts of medical interpreters' training and practice. They are mentioned throughout this book and our medical interpreter training course is aligned with these organizations.

ABOUT THE ACADEMY OF INTERPRETATION

The Academy of Interpretation www.academyofinterpretation.com is a learning platform that expands access to educational offerings and establishes a standard of quality in the language services industry. We aim to professionalize the language services industry through proper training and credentialing. The Academy believes that interpreters are crucial to our communities and that we want to recognize their contributions by providing them with the tools for proper performance.

COURSE EXPECTATIONS (CONTINUED FROM SYLLABUS)

This is an intensive course; if you have other time-consuming commitments you will need to take care of on the same days as this course, you should consider re-scheduling your other commitments or withdrawing from the course.

Note: If taking online version, disregard statement above, as this course is also taught in person. The online version is self-paced.

At the end of this course, you should be able to successfully perform all the objectives listed in the Course Syllabus. These skills cannot be learned passively, so you will need to play an active role in the exercises, role play practice sessions, and complete your homework before each day of class.

STUDENT EXPECTATIONS

Students may dress comfortably during the course, but the Academy of Interpretation reserves the right to modify dress standards as needed. Cellphones are permitted in the classroom, but trainers have authority to ban all cellphone use in the classroom if cellphones become a distraction. Please be responsible with cellphones and courteous to your trainer and classmates at all times.

This training is a safe space for students. A safe space (also known as a "brave space") is a place where students can express themselves without fear of rejection or judgment based on any part of their identity. Racist, homophobic, bigoted, or otherwise disparaging remarks will result in immediate removal from the classroom and, if necessary, enrollment withdrawal from the course.

During this course, students will give and receive constructive criticism through the critique analysis process. Many sections of the course will invite students to analyze and critique one another, or to the entire class, about other students' performance. Students should feel comfortable pointing out perceived mistakes and areas of improvement, so long as they also mention the positive aspects of the performance and focus on the performance, not the student.

NOTES

1

INTERPRETING

LEARNING GOAL

After successful completion of the Interpreting chapter, participants will be able to do the following:

► Define the concept of interpreting and identify the main goal of the interpreter.

LEARNING OBJECTIVES:

Using the above goal, participants should also be able to do the following upon successful completion of this chapter:

► Understand the concept of interpretation.
► Know the main responsibility of the medical interpreter.
► Identify the difference between the source and target language.

IMPORTANT TERMS AND WORDS

► Interpreting
► Message
► Preserve the meaning
► Social work
► Profession
► Autonomy
► Perception of favoritism

► Ethics
► Professional distance
► Neutral
► Source language
► Target language
► Speech
► Conscious

The word "interpret" may mean many different things in the English language depending on the context. For example, many museumgoers "interpret" art, and some dancers "interpret" music. However, in the context of this course, which is for spoken languages only, the concept **to interpret** refers specifically to the process of listening to and analyzing a message received in one language, then converting that same message and delivering it in another language, all while preserving its meaning.

WHAT INTERPRETING IS NOT

Sometimes when talking about interpreting, it can be useful to understand what interpreting is **NOT**. For example, interpreting is NOT social work. Many interpreters enter the profession out of a desire to help others, and interpreters do indeed help many people. However, interpreters help people by interpreting their messages, and respecting their autonomy. Interpreting is not about recommending or discouraging patients or providers about something not related to interpreting.

Interpreters are NOT patient representatives. Interpreters need to be careful to be as professional as possible to all parties to avoid the perception of favoritism (this will be covered more in the ethics section). Patients especially may wish to become closer with their interpreters. However, interpreters should always maintain a professional distance and be neutral to both sides. This can be challenging, but it is the only way that patients and providers can trust the interpreters to faithfully interpret their messages to one another.

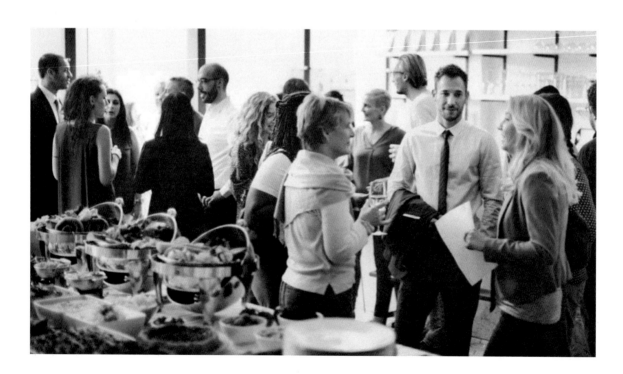

Personal closeness to patients (due to language and possibly culture) can cause unrealistic expectations from the patient's side as well as a level of mistrust from the provider's side (more on this later). Interpreting between languages can be confusing to discuss, so this textbook will introduce some common terms interpreters use when talking about interpreting.

> **Source language is the language that is to be interpreted or translated. Target language is the language in to which the source text or speech is to be translated or interpreted.**

The source and target language can vary during an interpreted conversation many times depending on who is speaking. Sometimes interpreting is unidirectional, such as when a presentation is interpreted from French into English. Other times, and mostly in healthcare, interpreting is 'dialogic', when a conversation, or 'dialogue' is interpreted in both directions. For example, if Yuanyuan and Arnold are a Mandarin speaker and a German speaker respectively, and neither person speaks the other's language, they could use an interpreter to understand one another. Whenever Yuanyuan is speaking Mandarin and the interpreter is interpreting Yuanyuan's messages, the source language is Mandarin, and the target language is German. However, whenever Arnold is speaking German and the interpreter is interpreting Arnold's message (which may be only a couple of seconds later), the source language is German, and the target language is Mandarin.

These terms are important because interpreters need to be conscious of errors that may occur when interpreting in either direction. *The interpreters' main goal is to enable understanding in communication between people who speak different languages.* The interpreter's goal is not to simply repeat words, but also to ensure that the messages are understood (IMIA Standards A-8 and A-9).

2

THE DIFFERENCE BETWEEN TRANSLATION AND INTERPRETATION

LEARNING GOAL

After successful completion of the difference between interpretation and translation chapter, participants will be able to do the following:

► Identify the difference between interpretation and translation

LEARNING OBJECTIVES:

Using the above goals, participants should also be able to do the following upon successful completion of this chapter:

► Differentiate between interpretation and translation.
► Know the needed skills for both interpretation and translation.

IMPORTANT TERMS AND WORDS

► Translation
► Interchangeably
► Professionals

► Rendering written text
► Signed message
► Skills

Many people use the two terms ***translation*** and ***interpretation*** interchangeably, which causes confusion among the public and the professionals, since there is a very clear difference between translation and interpretation.

The simplest way to differentiate between translation and interpretation is that translation means rendering written text materials from one language into another written form, while interpretation means rendering spoken or signed message from one language into another. Translation is written or typed. Interpretation is spoken or signed.

Many interpreters are not trained or qualified as translators, and many translators are not trained or qualified as interpreters. Interpreters and translators have a different set of skills.

TRANSLATORS vs INTERPRETERS

While both translators and interpreters transfer meaning between languages, there's a big difference between what they do and the skills they possess. This simple infographic will help you determine which type you need.

WRITE
It's simple: translators write...

SPEAK
...and interpreters speak.

DELAYED
Your final translation product will take days or longer

REAL-TIME
The final product is delivered instantly

TARGET LANGUAGE
Translators don't have to be conversationally fluent in their source language but must be in the target language

BOTH LANGUAGES
It's essential that interpreters are native or near native in both langauges

DICTIONARIES
Translators rely on numerous industry-specific resources

ON-THE-SPOT
When on the job, interpreters do not have consult dictionaries, glossaries, etc.

EXAMPLE: LEGAL CONTRACT
A contract is a common example of a translation product

EXAMPLE: BUSINESS MEETING
Conducting a meeting? You will need an interpreter!

NOTES

3

SPECIALIZATIONS AND FIELDS OF INTERPRETING

LEARNING GOAL

After successful completion of the Specialization and Fields of interpreting chapter, participants will be able to do the following:

► Identify the specialization and fields of interpreting and describe the community interpreting field.

LEARNING OBJECTIVES:

Using the above goals, participants should also be able to do the following upon successful completion of this chapter:

► Understand the differences between all of the Specialization and Fields of interpreting.
► Differentiate between the community interpreting field and other fields of interpreting.

IMPORTANT TERMS AND WORDS

► Specialization and Fields
► Communication
► Cultures
► Trade and diplomacy
► Conference interpreters
► Educational interpreting
► Conflict zone
► Diplomatic interpreting,

► Liaison interpreting,
► Business interpreting, Community interpreting
► Social service,
► Law enforcement
► Consecutive interpreting
► Modes of interpreting

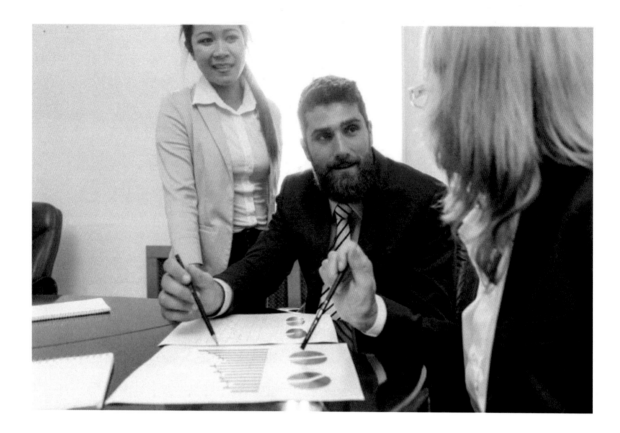

P rofessionals in many fields need interpreters because language and communication across cultures is essential in many fields. In some fields such as trade and diplomacy, interpreting has been around for hundreds or thousands of years old. In others, such as manufacturing, interpreting is fairly new because the need in that sector is more recent.

Today in the United States, medical, legal, and conference interpreters are the most well-known interpreting fields (specializations). However, there are many others emerging, such as educational interpreting and conflict zone interpreting. In this section, we explore diplomatic interpreting, liaison interpreting, business interpreting, and community interpreting (social service, law enforcement, and educational interpreting).

First, diplomatic interpreting occurs at large, prestigious bodies such as the United Nations and at minor-level diplomatic encounters. Consecutive interpreting (where the interpreter waits for a party to stop speaking before interpreting) is common in this sector. Diplomatic interpreting often needs to focus on and accurately convey nuances in meaning, including evasive answers and delicately crafted statements. Unlike in some interpreting specializations, where interpreters work for two parties, diplomats sometimes have an interpreter for each party, for political or security reasons.

Similar to diplomatic interpreting, liaison interpreting requires great flexibility.

Liaison interpreters need to be able and willing to move from location to location through tours, visits, and travel. In liaison interpreting, interpreters often use different modes of interpreting. Accomplished interpreters may use mobile interpreting equipment.

Third, business interpreting is a wide field that includes many sub-specialties. Business interpreters may be on calls between engineers discussing car specifications, a supplier and manufacturer, a wholesaler and a retailer, or different departments of a multi-national company. Business interpreters need to constantly be aware of how to position themselves in conference rooms to properly hear, control the flow of the conversation when necessary, and ensure conditions for optimal interpreting. One particular challenge for business interpreters is maintaining transparency in meetings or conference calls with many speakers.

Lastly, community interpreting is a catch-all term that includes different areas such as social service, healthcare, law enforcement, and educational interpreting. Community interpreting is often a relatively comfortable place for some interpreters; however, it requires a lot of practice. Just as there is a wide range of settings in community interpreting, there is also a wide range of ethical pitfalls into which unwary interpreters may fall.

4

MODALITY OF INTERPRETING

LEARNING GOAL

After successful completion of the Modality of interpreting chapter, participants will be able to do the following:

► Identify the three different Modalities of interpreting and describe the differences between in-person, telephonically, and via video modalities.

LEARNING OBJECTIVES:

Using the above goals, participants should also be able to do the following upon successful completion of this chapter:

► Understand the differences between in-person, telephonic, and video remote interpreting modalities.
► Distinguish between all of the three different modalities.
► Easily differentiate between spoken and signed communication.
► Identify the best-known modality of interpretation (On-Site Interpretation).
► Understand the impact of COVID-19 on interpreting and the increase need for remote interpretation (OPI and VRI).
► Identify the differences between the OPI and VRI.

IMPORTANT TERMS AND WORDS

- ► Modality of Interpreting
- ► On-Site Interpretation
- ► Face-to-face interpretation
- ► OPI
- ► VRI
- ► American Sign Language (ASL)

- ► Physical presence
- ► Telemedicine appointments
- ► LEP Limited English Proficient Patient
- ► Auditory interpretation
- ► COVID-19 Pandemic

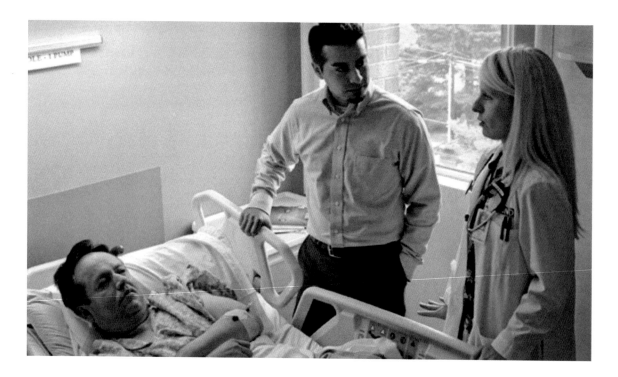

nterpreting can happen in-person, telephonically, or via video, but it must involve spoken or signed communication. In the United States, the most common form of signed communication is American Sign Language (**ASL**) and the most commonly-interpreted language pair is Spanish<>English.

In-person, telephonic, and video-remote interpreting are collectively known as **modalities** of interpreting. The best-known modality of interpretation is On-Site Interpretation; this involves traveling to the location where the person needs assistance and providing face-to-face interpretation.

There are also remote modalities of interpretation that do not require the physical presence of either one or all parties, such as Video Remote Interpretation (VRI), Over the Phone Interpretation (OPI) and interpreting for Telemedicine appointments when the three parties (LEP, provider and interpreter) are in different locations. VRI is a method in which an interpreter works from a computer with a camera and interprets through the screen. OPI is similar, except the interpreter will only provide auditory interpretation rather than being seen or seeing the person who needs interpretation services.

In 2020, due to the COVID-19 pandemic, there was a rise in the need and demand for remote interpreting modalities.

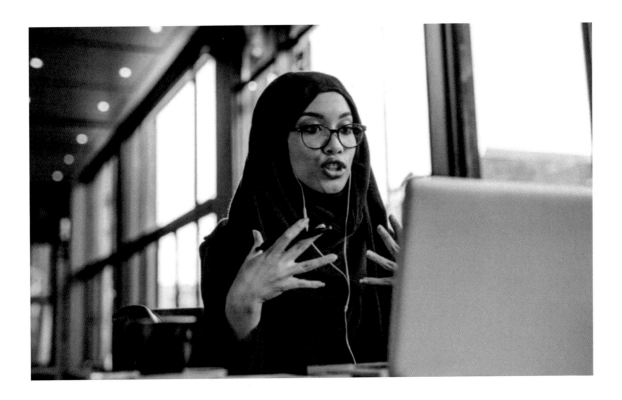

5

TYPES OF INTERPRETER EMPLOYMENT

LEARNING GOAL

After successful completion of the Types of Interpreter Employment chapter, participants will be able to do the following:

► Identify all types of interpreter employment and describe the nature job of medical, legal, business interpreters, and other types of interpreters.

LEARNING OBJECTIVES:

Using the above goals, participants should also be able to do the following upon successful completion of this chapter:

► Understand the differences between all types of interpreter employment.
► Distinguish between freelance interpreters, part-time interpreters, and full-time interpreters.
► Easily differentiate between spoken and signed communication.
► Identify the job of dual-role interpreters.
► Understand all of the differences between trained interpreters, Pro Bono interpreters, and ad-hoc interpreters.
► Understand the danger of using ad-hoc and non-trained interpreters for the safety of the patients and healthcare system.

IMPORTANT TERMS AND WORDS

- ► Subject matter
- ► Public facet
- ► Diverse backgrounds
- ► Deaf or hard of hearing people
- ► Legally entitled
- ► Part-time staff
- ► Employee benefits
- ► Freelance interpreters
- ► Independent contractors
- ► On-demand
- ► Decline assignments
- ► Paying clients

- ► Dual-role interpreters
- ► Bilingual
- ► Practicum interpreters
- Internship interpreters
- ► Volunteer interpreters
- ► Pro Bono interpreters
- ► Tax deductions
- ► Ad-hoc interpreter
- ► Interpreting competencies
- ► Ambiguity
- ► Federal courts
- ► High stakes settings

Professional interpretation is interpretation provided by a trained and tested individual who is competent to work in the subject matter at hand. It can be required in any professional or public facet of life that you can think of.

Interpretation is a huge part of living in a society with diverse backgrounds and cultures. Medical interpretation is needed at hospitals to interpret between providers and patients. Lawyers need legal interpreters to enable accurate communication with

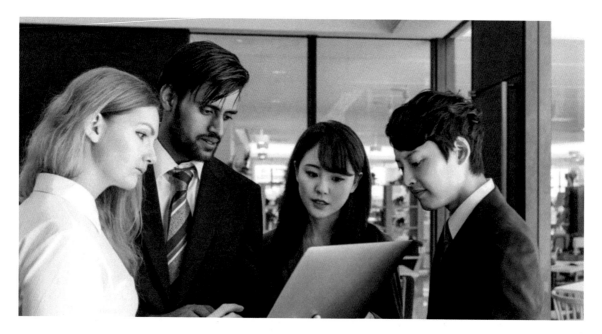

their clients, and potentially later in court. Businesses sometimes have foreign investors or customers who need interpretation services in order to communicate with them. Schools require interpreters for students who don't speak English as well as parents who have limited English proficiency. Deaf or hard of hearing people are legally entitled to an interpreter in any setting.

EMPLOYED INTERPRETERS work as full-time or part-time staff. They may be specialized in court/legal, diplomatic, government, or other type of interpreting. These interpreters have employee benefits, but they are not able to set their hours, nor can they accept or reject projects. They are usually paid by the hour or receive a weekly or monthly salary.

FREELANCE INTERPRETERS (also known as independent contractors) work on demand. Their work times, locations, and rates may vary. Freelance interpreters sell their work or services by the hour, day, job, etc., rather than working on a regular salary basis for one employer. They have the freedom to accept or decline assignments being offered to them, and usually work for many paying clients.

DUAL-ROLE INTERPRETERS are hired or employed professionals who are bilingual and have been trained and tested to be able to interpret professionally during their normal working hours. For example, a dual-role interpreter can be working as a nurse and be called to interpret as needed.

PRACTICUM INTERPRETERS (also known as internship interpreters) are those that are working towards a practice requirement for testing (certification) or the completion of a training. Practice professions typically have an internship component. In the business world, these are usually called internships, whereas in the medical sector these are called practicums.

VOLUNTEER INTERPRETERS are those that respond to requests for volunteers who can perform interpreting services, usually due to their concern for the individuals needing an interpreter (i.e. refugees, immigrants). These volunteers are commonly nonprofessional bilingual individuals who do not have any formal interpreter training. While many non-profits make requests to professional interpreters to volunteer their interpretation services for their conferences or meetings, the interpreting associations frown upon this type of interpreting as it undervalues and undercuts the professionalization of interpreting. Some organizations have set up their interpreting systems to rely solely on volunteer interpreters, often using a lack of funds as justification. However, these are the same organizations that have no hesitation in paying for other professional services, such as photography, videography, graphic design, and catering. So clearly, the issue is not a lack of funds but a lack of understanding that interpreting is a profession that people must train for and develop their skill in. Typically, these organizations do not verify the qualifications of their 'volunteers', which is a big concern given that they run many risks by relying on individuals of varied skill levels with no form of monitoring the quality of the interpretation or reporting complaints. These organizations also do not realize the potential risks they face should a wrong interpretation cause an unwanted outcome.

PRO BONO INTERPRETERS are professional interpreters who choose to select a cause or an organization to volunteer for, just as lawyers and teachers may do. This arrangement is different as the organization is not requesting the service. It is the interpreter who is offering to provide an added service for his or her own benefit, such as tax deductions, community service requirements, or their own self-development efforts.

NON-PROFESSIONAL INTERPRETING is interpreting being performed by individuals who are not trained or tested in the interpretation specialization they are practicing in. The CLAS Standards admonishes the inadequate and dangerous use of bilingual children or untrained individuals to aid in the communication of their parents or family members due to the risk to the parties involved. These individuals are often called 'interpreters', but they are not interpreting, as they have not been formally trained to interpret. They are simply relaying partial information back and forth to the best of their ability. Accurate interpretation is a learned skill.

AD-HOC INTERPRETER is a term often used to describe bilingual or multilingual individuals such as family members, friends, or dual-role employees who have not been trained or tested for their interpreting competency. However, since the term utilizes the word "interpreter" it confuses people into thinking the service is being provided by a qualified interpreter.

The use of ad-hoc interpreters in medical and healthcare settings can be dangerous for both patient safety and in terms of liability for the healthcare providers and the organizations and systems in which they work. Due to their lack of training and testing, ad-hoc interpreters can cause misunderstanding and miscommunication. Professional medical interpreters are more accurate.

Additionally, "asking people who have not received healthcare interpreter training to perform this task compromises some fundamental ethical aspects of healthcare between providers and patients." (California Standards for Healthcare Interpreters, 2002).

Healthcare providers and their staff should not rely on patient family and friends to interpret.

The use of ad-hoc interpreters can cause serious impediments to communication with patients and their families and patient safety and satisfaction will suffer.

NOTES

6

THE ROLES OF INTERPRETERS

LEARNING GOAL

After successful completion of The Roles of Interpreter's chapter, participants will be able to do the following:

► Identify all types of barriers to the communication between LEP (Limited-English Person) patients and the providers and be able to describe the different roles of medical interpreters in a medical encounter.

LEARNING OBJECTIVES:

Using the above goals, participants should also be able to do the following upon successful completion of this chapter:

► Identify the responsibilities of the interpreters and needed soft skills (Active Listening).
► Understand the mediation role of the interpreters and the meaning of the communication mediation.
► Understand the differences between the four roles of the medical interpreters (Conduit, Clarifier, Cultural Broker, and Patient Advocate roles).
► Differentiate between the different barriers to communication in the medical setting.
► Understand when interpreters can play the four different roles and which barrier requires the interpreters to have to switch from one role to another.
► Understand the role of the patient advocate and what the IMIA and NCIHC say about this role.

IMPORTANT TERMS AND WORDS

- Functions
- Tendency
- Conduit
- Linguistic conversion
- Non-thinking technicians
- Active listening skills
- Misconception
- Mediation role
- Monitor and arbiter
- Clarifier
- Intercultural mediator
- Patient Advocate
- Cultural representative
- Co-diagnostician
- Biomedical interpreter
- Intermediary
- Conciliator
- Cultural consultant
- Self-explanatory
- Role theories
- Maintaining flow
- Intervening
- Patient's history
- Pre-session
- Problem solving
- Resolve conflict

- Intercultural communication
- Empathetic listening
- Register Barrier
- Level of formality
- Specialized or technical language
- Facilitating communication
- Too colloquial (informal)
- A barrier of register
- Bipolar disorder
- Communication Barriers
- Environmental Barriers
- Inter-linguistic issues
- Intercultural Barriers
- Systemic discrimination barriers
- Racism,
- Discrimination
- Humiliation
- Ethnicity
- Race or sexual preference
- An ethical perspective
- Well-being
- Dignity
- The cultural proximity
- Offense
- An adversarial situation
- Practitioners

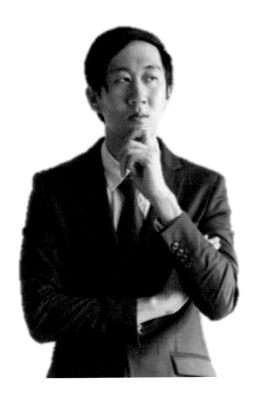

Now, we will cover the **roles of the interpreters**, or the functions that interpreters play in healthcare. Function can be further defined as the activity or purpose of a person.

There is a tendency among healthcare professionals to see the interpreter solely as a conduit, or a channel for linguistic conversion. This is verbalized by some people as speaking 'through' an interpreter. When a provider says, "please repeat what I say," or "tell her this," the provider may be under the impression that interpreters, like robots, or non-thinking technicians, merely repeat the same words or terms in another language (Hsieh, 2008). They do not realize that the interpreter, through active listening skills, must first gain complete understanding of

the message. Then, interpreters must reformulate the meaning of the message to successfully construct a new statement that conveys the exact intent and message of the original speaker. If the *meaning* of the original message uttered or signed is unclear, the interpreter will not be able to repeat it because repetition of words is not what he or she is doing in the first place. Since interpreters do not interpret words, but rather concepts and meaning between two cultures and languages, it may be more accurate to state that the interpreter's primary function is to mediate language and culture for mutual understanding. This is very different from repeating or telling someone something you heard in another language. Basically, stating that interpreters 'interpret' or 'convert' words from one language into another, enables this misconception to exist. The concept of interpreters having a mediation role is rarely on the provider's mind (Souza, 2016). We will discuss what is mediation is in a minute. But first, what specific roles have researchers described observing medical interpreters in?

Well, research on medical interpreters' role(s) has shown that a wide variety of roles exist including but not limited to: monitor and arbiter (Takeda, 2009), welcomer (Angelelli, 2004), conduit, clarifier, patient advocate, intercultural mediator (California Healthcare Interpreters Association, 2003), gatekeeper, informant, cultural representative, co-diagnostician (Hsieh, 2006), linguistic agent (Kelly, 2000), community agent, system agent (Leanza, 2005), cultural informant, biomedical interpreter (Kaufert & Koolage, 1984), intermediary, conciliator, cultural consultant (Raval, 2005), and intercultural mediator (Souza, 2016). There is still a need to further explore issues surrounding the role and responsibilities of medical interpreters within the contextualized framework of therapeutic communication goals. Although, now researchers are moving away from describing the profession as roles, and instead aim to describe the tasks and responsibilities of the interpreter to explain *what interpreters do,* versus *who they are* or act as.

These roles are mostly self-explanatory and clearly showcase the numerous kinds of functions that are fulfilled, or expected to be fulfilled, by a medical interpreter. When explaining the difference between Haitian Creole and French, the interpreter becomes a 'linguistic educator'. When explaining how to work with interpreters, he or she could be called a 'client educator'. However, the reality is that the only purpose of role theories and explanations is to enhance the understanding of the interpreter's work and strategies. They are not necessarily something that needs to be adhered to as a set of rules. Interpreters are interpreters and do not change roles, but simply take on different actions, which are sometimes described as roles.

Certain studies have showed that there can be conflict between some roles, or functions, such as 'maintaining flow' and 'intervening', which seem to be at odds with one another. This requires interpreters to constantly analyze next steps while interpreting (Shlesinger, 2002). Another common role conflict occurs when the patient wants the interpreter to take on the role of 'friend' and 'representative' or 'personal advocate', or when the provider wants the interpreter to be their 'clinical helper' by asking the interpreter to take the patient's history (instead of/for the provider). As you learn more about roles, you will see that these particular requests are not roles within the work of mediation. You will also learn that an interpreter can perform many roles or functions at the same time.

Interpreters should not think they are only working as interpreters when they are actively interpreting. Their job as an interpreter adjusts and switches between various roles and tasks during the entire process. From the arrival of an assignment to pre-session introductions, communication flow management, problem solving, intervening, and closure activities, the interpreter will be working and constantly utilizing different skills. The time an interpreter is interpreting is but a small portion of an interpreter's entire work, so the interpreting role cannot be limited to the interpretation time alone.

AN INTERPRETER IS A TYPE OF MEDIATOR, BUT WHAT IS A MEDIATOR?

There are many types of mediators. Most are familiar with conflict mediators, intermediaries hired to attempt to resolve conflict through moderate problem-solving until all parties arrive at an agreement. However, interpreters are not conflict mediators. Interpreters, especially dialogue interpreters (who interpret one-on-one back and forth conversations), are communication mediators. The difference is that they are not interpreting an adversarial relationship. Most medical interpreting sessions are collaborative, where the provider and the patient have the same goal in mind, which is the wellbeing of the patient.

WHAT IS MEANT BY 'COMMUNICATION' MEDIATION?

Interpreters mediate intercultural communication between people. Communication requires understanding. If one communicates a message but the listener did not understand, there was no communication, there was just the transfer of information. Therefore, language alone does not do the trick. Interpreters are not 'language' mediators because they are not mediating languages. They are mediating communication, which uses language to communicate. In intercultural communication, there are at least two languages, so the mediation is inter-linguistic and intercultural. Therefore,

from this perspective, one may conclude that interpreters are communication professionals. In addition to being communication professionals, interpreters are also language professionals, since they need to know at least two languages at a professional level of proficiency and know the art of linguistic interpretation in all modes. Of course, they are also interpreting professionals. However, remember that being an interpreter is not just about the role you perform when interpreting what other individuals state or sign.

The role of interpreting requires managing the communication, as a group facilitator does, in addition to performing interpretation during the communicative session. Communication mediators need to pay close attention to all facets of communication, such as their own communication, ensure understanding (IMIA, A-8), handle the dynamics of the students, such as managing the dynamics of the triad (IMIA A-11), intervene when necessary (IMIA, B-2), and much more.

Most mediators consider empathetic listening as one of their core skills, and this is especially relevant in therapeutic communication. In addition, the advanced skill of reframing is necessary in communication mediation. This involves reframing target messages, so they have the same effect as if stated in the source language. Whereas the mediation role is the overarching role of the interpreter, there are four roles that are the most popular when explaining medical interpreting, and these will be explained for this training's purposes.

THE FOUR ROLES

The four historic interpreter roles usually used in interpreter training will be described in this section. The four roles are 1) Conduit, 2) Clarifier, 3) Intercultural Mediator or Cultural Broker, and 4) Patient Advocate. Other interpreting courses may use different names for these roles, but the meaning is similar and the problems these roles address are the same.

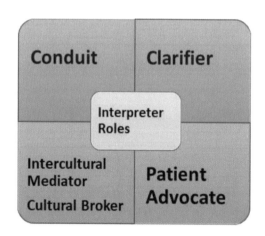

CHANGING ROLES

As stated before, interpreting what others state or sign is but one of the interpreter's tasks. The interpreter must be able to flow from role to role during the interpreted

session as potential misunderstandings arise and are resolved. *The most appropriate role for the interpreter is always the role that will ensure effective and accurate communication between the main parties involved.*

THE ROLE OF CONDUIT

As a Conduit, the interpreter is simply reframing the message from the source language to the target language and then restating or signing in the target language what the speaker said in the source language. In the Conduit role, the interpreter always interprets meaning for meaning.

> The Conduit role is the role in interpreting which only interpreters can perform and is the role which is viewed as the act of interpreting. Amongst the four roles, it is the only role that is not meant for problem solving.

The interpreter plays the conduit role when there is a linguistic barrier. For example, a patient may only speak the Arabic language while the provider may only speak the English language. The provider will ask some questions in English and the patient will answer in Arabic. However, because of the language barrier, the two of them cannot communicate with each other. This is when the interpreter steps in as a conduit to enable understanding between the patient and the provider by interpreting everything that is said faithfully and accurately.

THE ROLE OF CLARIFIER

Now that we have discussed the role of conduit, we will be talking about the other three roles, which all involve problem solving in some way. Problem solving may or may not require intervention (as you will see later). The role of **clarifier** is used to manage the flow of communication between two or more parties. Interpreters need to intervene in their own voice to direct the flow of communication. For example, if two people are speaking at once, the interpreter needs to state that he or she cannot interpret for more than one person at a time so that the two parties can be mindful of not speaking over each other. In this example, the interpreter is problem solving during a situation when something is making it too difficult for them to properly do their interpretation. Usually the interpreter plays the role of the clarifier when there is an issue related to the flow of the communication, the understanding of a message, or the meaning of a message. There could be a problem with hearing what was said, a problem with the message or length of sentences used, a problem with a difficult term, etc. These problems or challenges are sometimes called barriers and they must be removed and cleared to allow for accurate interpretation.

COMMUNICATION BARRIERS

REGISTER BARRIER refers to a misunderstanding due to a difference in the level of formality or complexity of language used between the communicating parties. A "register" is a linguistic term (further discussed in Section 15) referring to formal and informal, specialized or technical language choices speakers regularly make in conversation.

Medical interpreting is about facilitating communication and ensuring equal access to medical services. Therefore, register barriers are a key concern to interpreters. They occur when someone is using terms that are too complex or too colloquial (informal) for the other person to understand completely.

A barrier of register usually prompts the interpreter to play the role of clarifier to explain a complicated medical term or a term that does not have similarity in the target language. Interpreters need to be aware when the term being interpreted into the target language will confuse the patient because it might not transfer over when translated literally from the English language into the target language; for example, the medical term *Bipolar disorder* does not make sense when translated literally into the Arabic language. The interpreter must explain what this term means, using the clarifier role, rather than just acting as a conduit.

COMMUNICATION BARRIERS are barriers to understanding which can include: being unable to hear what was just said, being unable to interpret because someone is speaking too fast, or simply not being sure of the meaning of the message just uttered or signed. Additionally, a communication barrier can result from the difficulty of expressing a concept to be interpreted. For example, if the interpreter cannot think of an equivalent term to use for a concept stated in the source language, the interpreter may ask that party to rephrase or explain to make it easier to interpret. In doing this, the interpreter is intervening to identify and remove the communication barrier between the provider and the patient.

ENVIRONMENTAL BARRIERS are the barriers related to the space one is working in. For example, if the space the interpreter is interpreting in has no walls and is very noisy, this noise barrier may need to be removed by requesting to move to another place or to have all parties speak louder.

> As a clarifier, the interpreter helps ensure the removal of all these types of communication barriers so that complete and accurate interpretation can be provided.

Whereas keeping the flow of communication may seem to be the goal, managing the flow of communication is of utmost importance, as accuracy and completeness of interpretation is the most important

service the interpreter can provide. There is no benefit in glossing over possible misunderstandings or mistakes in interpretation in the name of keeping the illusion of a seamless flow of communication.

THE ROLE OF INTERCULTURAL MEDIATOR OR CULTURAL BROKER

Since language is a component of culture, inter-linguistic issues or barriers will include intercultural issues or barriers. The role of intercultural mediator or cultural broker is the same as that of clarifier, except in this case, it involves identifying and seeking interventions to remove intercultural barriers.

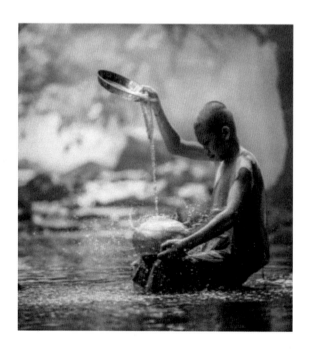

INTERCULTURAL BARRIERS are barriers that exist due to differences of cultural views, beliefs, traditions, or behaviors. These differences may cause misunderstandings. Therefore, interpreters need to be able to identify, inquire, and work to help the parties resolve these intercultural misunderstandings.

Take for example, the fact that some cultures use a workweek of Sunday through Thursday instead of Monday through Friday. This could cause confusion when someone is not familiar with this cultural difference. If a patient says, "the first day of the week", he or she may assume everyone knows they are referring to Sunday. However, if the interpreter simply interprets "the first day of the week" literally, the provider may think they are speaking about Monday. In this case, the interpreter should clarify if the patient is referring to a Sunday or Monday. The 'assumption' that the first day of the week is Monday is a cultural assumption, based on tradition and practices that could be thousands of years old.

> **Interpreters need to pay close attention to properly identify an issue as a cultural issue.**

Whereas the interpreter may think that the issue is cultural, it could simply be a case of missing information, or an issue of a patient's personal opinion. Therefore, the interpreter should be careful not to make any assumptions, and instead ask the speaker questions to confirm that the issue is indeed the result of a cultural misunderstanding. For example, a female patient might refuse a certain male provider and the interpreter might assume that the patient refused the male provider because of gender, and because the patient comes from a very conservative culture. When in fact, the patient does not like this provider because she thinks that the provider is not good, and he will not be able to help her as she wishes. In this example, the interpreter should not assume anything. The interpreter must first confirm what he thinks with the patient, before the interpreter reinforces a gender stereotype and makes a wrong assumption.

THE ROLE OF PATIENT ADVOCATE

Lastly, interpreters sometimes need to adopt a role called patient advocate.

This role is mostly used to remove **systemic** discrimination **barriers**, which are differences in beliefs that lead to unjust treatment (*e.g.* racism, discrimination, humiliation) of patients based on their identity (gender, age, ethnicity, race or sexual preference).

Some language services and providers have strict rules about the patient advocate role and advise their interpreters not to play this role. Although interpreters should remember that NOT acting and playing the role of a patient advocate when seeing systemic discrimination occur may be putting the interpreter at risk of being accused of participating in such an act of discrimination. Therefore, sometimes the interpreters must do something to help from an ethical perspective. However, this does not necessarily need to occur during the communicative event. It all depends on the situation as will be explained in the next section.

WHAT DO THE IMIA AND NCIHC HAVE TO SAY ABOUT PATIENT ADVOCACY?

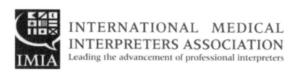

INTERNATIONAL MEDICAL INTERPRETERS ASSOCIATION
Leading the advancement of professional interpreters

National Council on Interpreting in Health Care

Neither the IMIA nor the NCIHC explicitly use the term patient advocacy. Instead, they refer to the advocacy role as a role to represent one of the parties when the behavior of the other is detrimental to the well-being or dignity of that individual, be it the patient, the provider, or another person in the communicative session. While the IMIA does not use the term advocacy in its standards, it does state that "the cultural proximity of the patient with the interpreter may cause the patient to want the interpreter to act as his or her advocate". Regarding the patient advocacy role, it states the following in the ethical section of its standards:

Interpreters deal with discrimination (IMIA: C-7). It further states that, "On occasions where the interpreter feels strongly that either party's behavior is affecting access

to or quality of service, or compromising either party's dignity, [the interpreter] uses effective strategies to address the situation. If the problem persists, [the interpreter] knows and uses institutional policies and procedures relevant to discrimination". **Related IMIA Ethical Principle:** Interpreters will engage in patient advocacy only when appropriate and necessary for communication purposes, using professional judgment.

NCIHC states the following in its Standards of Practice:

ADVOCACY: To prevent harm to parties that the interpreter serves. The interpreter may speak out to protect an individual from serious harm. For example, an interpreter may intervene on behalf of a patient with a life-threatening allergy, if the condition has been overlooked. The interpreter may advocate on behalf of a party or group to correct mistreatment or abuse. For example, an interpreter may alert his or her supervisor to patterns of disrespect towards patients. *Related ethical principle*: When the patient's health, well-being or dignity is at risk, an interpreter may be justified in acting as an advocate.

Note that both standards apply the advocacy role as a response to either party's behavior, not just the provider's behavior towards the patient. Even in cases of discrimination, we cannot assume that the discrimination will be against the patient. There are cases where patients discriminate against providers.

Lastly, it is important for interpreters to realize that accusing someone of acts of discrimination or offense towards another party is a serious issue that may cause repercussions to the individual and to the interpreter. It is important that the interpreter be certain and not use the discrimination card when it is perhaps simply a situation of a difficult interpersonal relationship between the provider and the patient. The interpreter needs to know the protocols in place where they work, and their first line of action may be to discuss the issue with a supervisor after the communicative event, and not during it. Only very skilled interpreters with high levels of diplomatic skills should consider advocacy during the interpretation, as it can become an adversarial situation to the detriment of all the parties involved. Interpreter training usually includes techniques to address mild forms of discrimination.

IN SUMMARY

The role of the interpreter encompasses a much broader scope than the actual act of interpreting or the four roles described in this section. Researchers ultimately consider medical interpreters as practitioners (Dean & Pollard, 2005), engaged in a practice profession, like medicine, law, teaching, counseling, or law enforcement, where careful consideration and judgment regarding situational and human interaction factors are central to doing effective work.

One can contrast the practice professions with the technical professions, such as engineering and accounting, where knowledge and skills pertaining to the technical elements of a job are largely sufficient to allow the professional to produce a competent work product. Interpreters function more like practice professionals than technicians due to the significance of situational and human interaction factors on their ultimate work product; that is, factors beyond the technical elements of the source and target language (Dean & Pollard, 2001; Gish, 1987; Humphrey & Alcorn, 1995; Metzger, 1999; Roy, 2000a; Wadensjo, 1998).

Interpreters cannot deliver effective professional service armed only with their technical knowledge of the source and target languages, culture, and a code of ethics. Like all practice professionals, they must supplement their technical knowledge and skills with input, exchange, and judgment regarding the providers and patients they are serving in a specific environment and in a specific communicative situation.

7

CONVERSION

LEARNING GOAL

- ► After successful completion of the Conversion chapter, participants will be able to do the following:
- ► Analyze and explain how to convert from English to the target language and vice versa.

LEARNING OBJECTIVES:

Using the above goals, participants should also be able to do the following upon successful completion of this chapter:

- ► Understand the fundamental work of any interpreter: expressing what someone says in one language in another language.
- ► Identify and explain the term: communicative autonomy.
- ► Interpret the message accurately and completely by applying the conversion concept.
- ► Identify the common motto of accuracy ("Add nothing, omit nothing, change nothing").
- ► Analyze the units of meaning to be accurate and complete.
- ► Understand when they can change the words and how they can do that.

IMPORTANT TERMS AND WORDS

- ► Communicative autonomy
- ► Fundamental
- ► Blunt
- ► Offensive
- ► Faithful rendition
- ► Operating table
- ► Critical
- ► Conjugation

- ► Mammals
- ► Ritual phrases
- ► Emergency Department
- ► Idioms
- ► The tip of the iceberg
- ► Undress
- ► Ache

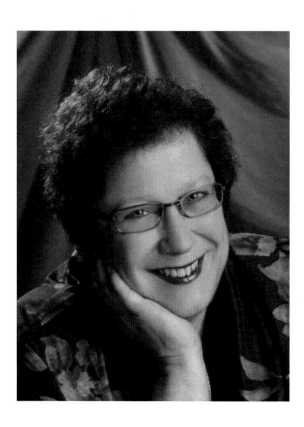

THE HEART OF INTERPRETING, BY CINDY ROAT

Hello there. My name is Cindy Roat. I'm a consultant and trainer of interpreters for healthcare settings. Today I'd like to introduce you to what is the fundamental work of any interpreter: expressing what someone says in one language in another language. This is called "conversion."

In the course of doing this, we want to support something we call communicative autonomy—hey, that's a fancy phrase! What does it mean?

To answer that question, let me ask another:

Who gets to decide WHAT is said in an interpreted conversation?

Does the speaker decide?

Does the interpreter decide?

If you said the speaker, you're right. The speaker chooses what he or she wants to say. The interpreter doesn't get to change the message in any way. That's communicative autonomy. "Autonomy" means independence, or freedom of action. So as interpreters, we support speakers' freedom to communicate whatever and however they want to. We make it possible for the speaker to be understood on their own terms.

You might say that we are the bridge over the language gap that helps two people who don't speak the same language communicate as if they did.

So, what if we do not like the message. Can we change it?

Nope.

But what if the speaker is too blunt?

Nope.

But what if the speaker is offensive?

Nope.

But what if we know that the speaker is actually lying?!

Well, that is the speaker's right. An English speaker could do all these things, and we support the right of the non-English speaker to do the same. We are there to make sure their message can be understood by the listener, just as the speaker said it. It is the speaker's right to be blunt, offensive, confusing—or even to lie.

The bottom line is that as interpreters, we follow these three simple rules:

Add nothing.

Omit nothing.

Change nothing.

This is the heart of accuracy. And accuracy is the heart of interpreting. If we are not accurate, nobody will trust that what we say is a faithful rendition of what the speaker said. So, we have to be absolutely accurate in our interpreting.

So, if the provider says, *"We did everything we could, but we couldn't save your husband. He died on the operating table. I'm sorry.",* that's what we interpret.

If the patient says, *"You are a terrible doctor! I'm going to sue you!"* that's what we interpret.

Add nothing.

Omit nothing.

Change nothing.

This sounds easy. Let's take a closer look.

If the provider says, *"What brings you in today?",* how will you interpret that?

If you can't add, omit or change anything, do you just convert the words into your non-English language?

What brings you in today?

What do you think? Try interpreting this word-for-word into your non-English language. Does it make sense?

Most likely not! Language doesn't work that way. Part of the beauty of languages is that they are all organized in different ways.

They put words in different orders, for example. In some languages, like English, the order of the words is critical. Sentences almost always go Subject, Verb, Object. So, the dog saw the tree is not the same as the tree saw the dog. But in Japanese, for example, a particle is added to the end of every word to show what role it plays in the sentence. So "dog tree saw" is the same as "tree dog saw." And the verb comes at the end.

In some languages, certain words are understood without being said. In Spanish, for example, the subject of a sentence is indicated by the conjugation of the verb. "I am" can be "Yo soy", but since "soy" is only used as the first-person present tense of the verb "to be", the "Yo" is understood and often dropped.

Another example of linguistic difference is how time is indicated. In English, the verb is conjugated to indicate time: I go, I will go, I went. In Mandarin Chinese, on the other hand, the verb in these three sentences would be the same. Time is indicated using specific time words, like "today," "now," "tomorrow".

We want the listener to understand the speaker. So, the interpretation we give in the listener's language has to sound natural and make sense in that language! We may need to leave some words out, add some words in, change the order...

"Wait a minute!", I hear you cry!

What happened to, "Add nothing, omit nothing, change nothing? You're breaking your own rules!"

Well, yes, I would be—if we were interpreting words.

But—**and this is very important—interpreters do not interpret words. We interpret MEANING.**

So, let's look at our doctor's utterance again.

"What brings you in today?"

What is the provider really asking? Whether the patient took the bus?

No, we understand that the provider is asking what the patient wants to talk to the doctor about. Why is the patient there?

So, an accurate interpretation might be *"What problem did you want to talk to me about today?"* or *"Why did you come in today?"*

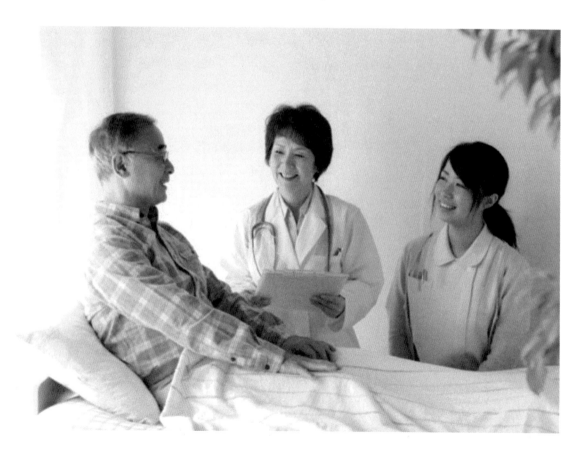

There's nothing about "bringing" at all. We have changed the words in order to be faithful to the meaning.

So, the real first rules of interpreting are:

···

Add no meaning. Omit no meaning. Change no meaning.

···

Here's another example. What if the nurse says,

"Did you have any trouble getting in today? It's raining cats and dogs out there!"

Or what if the doctor says,

"We've stabilized his condition, but he's not out of the woods yet."

Is the nurse saying that small mammals are falling from the sky? Is the doctor saying that the patient is somewhere lost in the woods? No, of course not. The nurse is saying that it's raining really hard, and she's just using a colorful expression to say it. A good interpretation would be,

"It's raining really hard." Not a dog or cat mentioned.

And the doctor is saying that the patient is still at risk. One possible rendering would be,

"He's still in some danger." No woods.

Did we change something? Yes, we changed the words, in order to conserve the meaning.

Let's look at this more carefully.

Some of what we interpret are ritual phrases. We say, "good morning." Is it really a good morning? It doesn't matter. The MEANING in this is that this is a polite greeting. What would be a polite greeting in your non-English language? The word for "morning" doesn't have to appear, just the greeting.

Here's another: "Thank goodness." It's an expression of relief. The most accurate conversion into your non-English language might not use the words "thank" or "good-ness." Because we're not interpreting words, we're interpreting...

(If you didn't say "meaning", go back to the beginning of Section 7 and start over!)

A final ritual phrase we use a lot in English: "Have a nice day." It's a polite way to end a conversation and to say good-bye. What would be the equivalent in your non-English language?

At other times, the source speech can only be understood in context.

Consider this statement by a nurse in the Emergency Department: *"We're going to move her onto the floor."* In the context of the ED, we know that this means that the patient will be admitted to the hospital when she is stable. If the context were, say, an EMT talking about a patient who has collapsed over a chair, the statement might have a different meaning.

Or this one, often heard in health care: "The tests were negative." In context, we know that this means that the tests did not find what they were looking for. In a different context—in a school, for example—this statement might have a different meaning.

Then there are idioms, like "raining cats and dogs."

"Runs in the family" indicates a characteristic shared by lots of family members; it has nothing to do with running.

"A piece of cake" means something's easy; it includes no pastries at all.

"The tip of the iceberg" is a small part of something much bigger, but involves no ice.

And how would you render "cutie-pie"?!!!

In all these cases, we interpret meaning, not words, so:

"People in the same family often get this same illness."

"Taking blood will be easy."

"We're afraid that this is just a small part of something much bigger."

"You are adorable/cute/lovely/endearing/charming…"

Sometimes, it can be hard to know exactly what the speaker meant.

Consider this question: *"When you left on your trip, did you take your pills?"*

Now, did the speaker mean to ask whether the patient took the pills with him in his suitcase when he went on his trip, or whether he swallowed his pills before he left?

We can't tell which of the two meanings was intended, neither from the statement nor the context. And since we are interpreting—what? Yes, MEANING—we cannot interpret something whose meaning we don't understand.

So, what do we do? We ask the speaker for clarification. More on that later.

Here's another example: The patient says, in Spanish, *"Tengo cinco hermanos."*

"Hermanos" can mean brothers, but it can also mean siblings—that is, brothers and sisters. Which did the patient mean? We don't know, so we need to ask for clarification.

If we are going to focus on meaning, not words, it makes sense to practice identifying what we call "units of meaning." For example, the question, *"What is your name?"* really has only one unit of meaning: "your name?"

The next question, though:

"I need your name, address, and home number" has 3 units of meaning: name, address, phone number. If we leave one out, we're omitting. If we mention social security number, we're adding. If we ask for the name, address, and shoe size, we've changed the meaning.

How about this one:

"Please undress and put on this gown. The doctor will be in shortly."

There are four units of meaning here:

Undress.

Put on the gown.

The doctor is coming.

The doctor will be here soon.

As long as we include these four units of meaning, we are being accurate. If we leave one out, if we add something else, or if we change one of the four, our interpretation is inaccurate.

Let's look at some examples of what a poor rendition might look like. Suppose a patient says this:

"It isn't so much a pain as a discomfort in my chest. A pressure, after I eat. Well, maybe it is a pain."

What are the units of meaning?

It isn't pain.

It's discomfort.

It's in my chest.

It's a pressure.

It's after I eat.

Maybe it is a pain.

So, here's one accurate rendition: *"It isn't really pain. It's more like discomfort, like a pressure in my chest after I eat. Well, I guess it really is pain."*

All the units of meaning, nothing added, nothing left out, nothing changed.

What would a rendition with an addition look like?

"It isn't really pain. It's more like discomfort, like a pressure in my chest after I eat. Sort of like indigestion. Well, I guess it really is pain."

Oops. That's not accurate. The patient never mentioned indigestion.

Now, how about if there were an omission?

"It isn't really pain. It's more like discomfort, like a pressure after I eat. Well, I guess it really is pain."

Hey, what happened to the reference to the chest? That could be important. This rendition is also inaccurate.

Here's a change in meaning.

"It isn't really pain. It's more like discomfort, like an ache in my chest then going down my arm. Well, I guess it really is pain."

If we used this rendition, the doctor might think that this patient's digestive problem is a heart attack. Accuracy is so important!

And by the way, there's another way that we can be inaccurate as interpreters, and that is by creating a rendition that doesn't sound natural in the target language—that puts the words in the wrong order, that uses the wrong grammar or that makes mistakes with vocabulary.

"Is not real pain. Is uncomfort, when I eat is like a pushing here."

These errors are usually signs that we need to improve our language skills in the language into which we are interpreting.

Accurate interpreting depends on understanding the meaning of what was said and then reproducing all the units of meaning without adding any, leaving any out, or changing any, ending up with a rendition that sounds natural in the target language.

Sound easy?

It's easy to do poorly, which is why lots of people think that anyone who is bilingual can interpret. But it's actually hard to be completely accurate. Even experienced professional interpreters are always honing their skills to become more accurate.

....

So next, we're going to do a series of exercises to get us thinking like interpreters.

....

8

THE FOUR MODES OF INTERPRETING

LEARNING GOAL

After successful completion of The Four Modes of Interpreting chapter, participants will be able to do the following:

► Define the four different modes of interpreting and explain the differences between all of them.

LEARNING OBJECTIVES:

Using the above goals, participants should also be able to do the following upon successful completion of this chapter:

► Understand and explain the difference between modes of interpreting and roles of interpreters.
► Fully understand the differences between all four modes of interpreting; consecutive, simultaneous, sight translation and summarization.
► Identify the default mode of interpreting in the healthcare setting; consecutive.
► Explain when they have to use the simultaneous mode of interpreting.
► Understand when they have to summarize the messages.

IMPORTANT TERMS AND WORDS

► Modes of interpreting
► Methods
► Controversial topic
► Circumstances
► Functions

► The IMIA Standard
► Legitimate need
► Decalage
► Trauma
► Verbalizing

Consecutive Interpreting	Simultaneous Interpreting	Sight Translation	Summerization

Now that we have briefly talked about some terms used in interpreting, it is time to describe the ways in which interpreting is performed. Which are **methods** and which are **modes** of interpreting, is a controversial topic in the field of interpreting. For the purposes of this training, the Academy of Interpretation describes the four types of interpreting performance as modes.

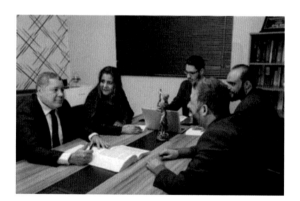

The **modes of interpreting** describe the methods of performance an interpreter can utilize to deliver an interpretation into a target language. Interpreters use different modes of interpreting under different circumstances. The four modes of interpreting are consecutive, simultaneous, sight translation, and summarization.

Interpreters should be careful not to confuse modes (*eg.* consecutive and simultaneous) with roles. Interpreters can remember that modes are the *methods* of interpretation, while roles are mostly the *functions* interpreters perform or the roles they play to do their work.

CONSECUTIVE INTERPRETING

CONSECUTIVE INTERPRETING is when the interpreter interprets after the speaker stops speaking. The speaker usually says a few words, a phrase, or a few sentences, and then waits for the interpreter to interpret before continuing. Consecutive interpreting is sometimes known as "pause" interpreting because the speaker pauses to wait for the interpretation of what was said.

> Consecutive interpreting is by far the most common mode in medical interpreting, and it is the most accurate mode of interpreting for most interpreters.

According to the IMIA Standard, the interpreter uses the mode that best

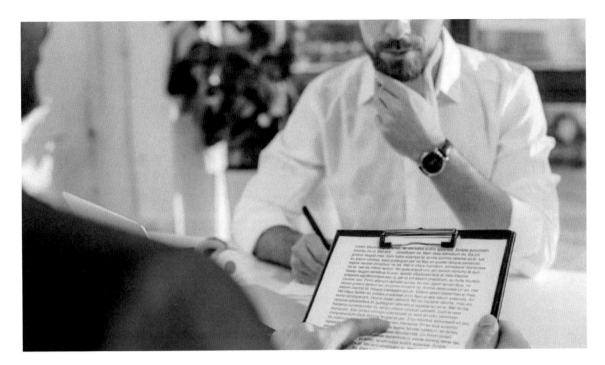

enhances comprehension and least interrupts the speaker's train of thought, given the demands of the situation, and that that best preserves accuracy (IMIA, A-5, A&B)

When in an interpreting session, it can be tempting to switch to another mode of interpreting; however, interpreters should stay in consecutive in most situations unless there is a legitimate need to switch (described in detail in the next section).

It is the professional interpreter's decision which mode to use and when.

SIMULTANEOUS INTERPRETING

In simultaneous interpreting, the interpreter interprets while the speaker is speaking, with a slight delay, called decalage. This mode is most commonly used in legal or conference settings. This mode is used when it is inappropriate or impossible to have a speaker pause.

This may happen in the following circumstances:

► There is not enough time

► The provider is giving a presentation or explanation to several parties

► Group therapy sessions

► Pediatric interpreting (interpreting the patient-provider conversation simultaneously to the parent)

► Inpatient resident visits (interpreting resident-doctor conversation simultaneously for the patient)

One of the more common situations where interpreters switch to simultaneous mode is when a patient is describing a traumatic event he or she experienced.

Many times, describing that trauma is itself a traumatic experience for the patient.

If interpreters find that the patient cannot pause at brief intervals after several requests, the interpreter should consider switching to simultaneous mode for the important messages not to be lost.

SIGHT TRANSLATION

SIGHT TRANSLATION is when an interpreter reads a text written in one language (the source language) and interprets it by verbalizing or signing the messages into another language (the target language). The interpreter does not provide a written translation of the document in question.

Ideally, parties would always translate important documents in advance of the interpreting session; however, this is often not the case. Interpreters should be careful to ensure that they only sight translate documents that are **short** in length. This is because any document that is longer than two pages should be translated for the patient. Interpreters should feel comfortable declining to sight translate a document that requires further preparation or terminology research (discussed in detail in the Sight Translation sections of this training).

SUMMARIZATION

SUMMARIZATION occurs when the interpreter summarizes the source language message into another language. Summarization is a difficult task as it requires the interpreter to analyze which units of meaning are most important. For example, usually adjectives and adverbs may be omitted if they are not central to the message. Usually summarization is requested by the provider. It is important to note that anything that is to be sight translated needs to be done completely, without omissions. If the provider asks the interpreter to summarize the consent or discharge instructions, or to interpret the provider's summary, the interpreter must sign at the bottom that a summary of what is rendered in the document was interpreted, and not the entire text in the document.

Interpreters sometimes need to resort to summarization when they are unable to interpret the entire messages that a speaker stated. This may be because the speaker spoke for too long, there was a distraction, the interpreter did not fully understand the speaker, or for some other reason.

Once again, if an interpreter uses summarization as a performance method, it is important that the interpreter disclose that the rendition is a summarization.

> Summarization should always be a last resort for interpreters using consecutive and simultaneous modes. Interpreters should not summarize sight translations for patient for safety reasons. However, sometimes providers request a summarization sight translation of a patient's medical records. Always disclose or document summarization to all parties for transparency.

NOTES

9

THE CODE OF ETHICS FOR INTERPRETERS IN HEALTH CARE

LEARNING GOAL

After successful completion of The Code of Ethics for Interpreters in Health Care chapter, participants will be able to do the following:

► Define and apply the code of ethics for interpreters in the healthcare setting.

LEARNING OBJECTIVES:

Using the above goals, participants should also be able to do the following upon successful completion of this chapter:

► Understand and explain the necessity of the code of ethics for interpreters.
► Know that the code of ethics are not morals.
► Fully understand that the ethics exist to help interpreters make decisions when faced with a difficult ethical situation.
► Understand that there are two well-known code of ethics for medical interpreters; NCIHC Code of Ethics and IMIA Code of Ethics.
► Understand and be able to explain the NCIHC Code of Ethics.
► Realize what partiality looks like.

IMPORTANT TERMS AND WORDS

- Codes of ethics
- Potential pitfalls
- Morals
- Individual beliefs
- Preferences
- Mandatory
- Definitive
- Dilemmas
- Credentials
- Breaches
- Mediate communication
- NATIONAL STANDARDS OF PRACTICE
- Ethical principle
- Spirit of the message
- Cultural context
- Substituting
- Redundant
- Irrelevant
- Relevant requirements
- Maintains confidentiality
- Disclose information

- Patient's consent
- Interpreter bias
- Inherent dignity
- Encounter
- Cultural Awareness
- Biomedical culture
- Potential conflict
- Surgery consent form
- Discredit
- Novice interpreters
- Life-threatening allergy
- Emotionally detached
- Impartial stance
- Therapeutic rapport
- Professionalism
- Impartiality
- Demeanor
- Faithfulness and fidelity
- Literal interpretation
- Debrief

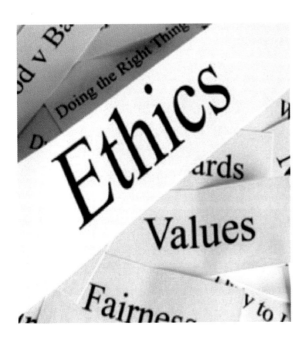

Interpreting is a complex task with many potential pitfalls (areas where mistakes are easy and common). The best way to avoid interpreting pitfalls is to know about them and learn the solutions. Some of those pitfalls and solutions are covered within our discussion of ethics here.

The codes of ethics exist to help interpreters make decisions about what to do, especially in difficult situations. They represent a set of guidelines that help interpreters perform their work in the most effective way possible.

ETHICS ARE NOT MORALS

It is easy to confuse the things an interpreter should do professionally with the things that an interpreter might think are inherently "right" or "wrong;" however, professional **ethics** are not morals; they are standards agreed upon by the profession.

A person's understanding of what is appropriate and inappropriate may guide that person in making the right personal decisions. However, professional ethical rules are to be followed by all professionals.

Interpreter ethics are simply the broad rules that help interpreters know what is appropriate and what is inappropriate when interpreting. These ethics are shared by the whole interpreting profession, and they are independent from an individual interpreter's beliefs.

Instead of relying on individual beliefs and preferences of what is acceptable (a varying standard based on personal opinion), a code of ethics provides a list of standards that interpreters should use to hold themselves and each other accountable.

(Adapted from the 2014 **Bridging the Gap: Medical Interpreter Training** *presentation by* **Cross Cultural Health Care Program***).*

ETHICS ARE MANDATORY

Ethics exist to help interpreters make decisions when faced with a difficult ethical situation. A code of ethics is not a definitive "how to" solve all the difficult dilemmas faced by an interpreter, but rather a set of rules to follow and use as a guideline to avoid behaving in a way that could harm the interpreter, the provider, the patient or the profession.

Ethics are not mere suggestions. They are mandatory principles that all interpreters should follow to maintain trust for the interpreting profession and to help both providers and patients. Certified medical or healthcare interpreters, for instance, may lose their national certification credentials due to breaches in the code of ethics.

....

ALWAYS REMEMBER: The basic purpose of the interpreter is to mediate communication between patient and provider, by interpreting everything that is said accurately and completely, as well as problem solving and intervening when necessary in order to ensure accurate communication.

....

Interpreters interpret messages, not words! Interpreters should not *add messages, omit messages,* or *change messages* conveyed, even though this may mean omitting words, adding terms, or changing terminology in order to communicate the same message into another language. Interpreters should also problem solve and intervene when necessary.

The most well-known code of ethics for medical interpreters are:

1. NCIHC Code of Ethics (see: https://www.ncihc.org/assets/documents/NCIHC National Code of Ethics.pdf)

2. IMIA Code of Ethics (see: https://www.imiaweb.org/code & https://www.imiaweb.org/uploads/pages/376_2.pdf)

Each organization has the code and explanatory text. Here are the code tenets of both organizations:

1. A NATIONAL CODE OF ETHICS FOR INTERPRETERS IN HEALTH CARE, https://www.ncihc.org/assets/documents/publications/NCIHC National Code of%20Ethics.pdf)

2. IMIA Code of Ethics & IMIA Guide on Medical Interpreter Ethical Conduct, https://www.imiaweb.org/code & https://www.imiaweb.org/uploads/pages/376_2.pdf

The codes of ethics don't give definitive answers for every single situation; instead, they use generalized rules to represent the shared goals, values, and expectations for the members of a profession.

THE NATIONAL STANDARDS OF PRACTICE FOR INTERPRETERS IN HEALTH CARE
....

We will cover the NATIONAL STANDARDS OF PRACTICE for Interpreters in Health Care in our course because it is the national standards of practice for medical interpreters. However, we will also include other codes of ethics and standards of practice that have been created by other professional organizations or state professional organizations.

The NATIONAL STANDARDS OF PRACTICE for Interpreters in Health Care was generously funded by The Commonwealth Fund and The California Endowment.

STANDARDS OF PRACTICE ACCURACY

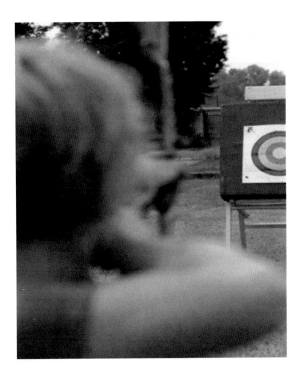

OBJECTIVE: To enable other parties to know precisely what each speaker has said.

RELATED ETHICAL PRINCIPLE: Interpreters strive to render the message accurately, conveying the content and spirit of the original message, taking into consideration the cultural context.

► The interpreter renders all messages accurately and completely, without adding, omitting, or substituting. For example, an interpreter repeats all that is said, even if it seems redundant, irrelevant, or rude.

► The interpreter replicates the register, style, and tone of the speaker.

For example, unless there is no equivalent in the patient's language, an interpreter does not substitute simpler explanations for medical terms a provider uses, but may ask the speaker to re-express themselves in language (words) more easily understood by the other party.

► The interpreter advises parties that everything said will be interpreted. For example, an interpreter may explain the interpreting process to a provider by saying "everything you say will be repeated to the patient."

► The interpreter manages the flow of communication. For example, an interpreter may ask a speaker to pause or slow down.

► The interpreter corrects errors in interpretation. For example, an interpreter who has omitted an important word corrects the mistake as soon as possible.

► The interpreter maintains transparency. For example, when asking for clarification, an interpreter says to all parties, "I, the interpreter, did not understand, so I am going to ask for an explanation."

CONFIDENTIALITY

OBJECTIVE: To honor the private and personal nature of the health care interaction and maintain trust among all parties.

RELATED ETHICAL PRINCIPLE: Interpreters treat as confidential, within the treating team, all information learned in the performance of their professional duties, while observing relevant requirements regarding disclosure.

▶ The interpreter maintains confidentiality and does not disclose information outside the treatment team, except with the patient's consent or if required by law. For example, an interpreter does not discuss a patient's case with family or community members without the patient's consent.

▶ The interpreter protects written patient information in his or her possession. For example, an interpreter does not leave notes on an interpreting session in public view.

IMPARTIALITY

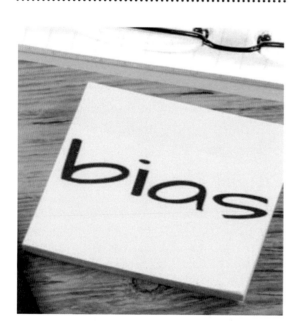

OBJECTIVE: To eliminate the effect of interpreter bias or preference.

RELATED ETHICAL PRINCIPLE: Interpreters strive to maintain impartiality and refrain from counseling, advising, or projecting personal biases or beliefs.

▶ The interpreter does not allow personal judgments or cultural values to influence objectivity.

    ▫ For example, an interpreter does not reveal personal feelings through words, tone of voice, or body language.

▶ The interpreter discloses potential conflicts of interest, withdrawing from assignments if necessary. For example, an interpreter avoids interpreting for a family member or close friend.

RESPECT

OBJECTIVE: To acknowledge the inherent dignity of all parties in the interpreted encounter.

RELATED ETHICAL PRINCIPLE: Interpreters treat all parties with respect.

▶ The interpreter uses professional, culturally appropriate ways of showing respect. For example, in greetings, an interpreter uses appropriate titles for both patient and provider.

► The interpreter promotes direct communication among all parties in the encounter. For example, an interpreter may tell the patient and provider to address each other, rather than the interpreter.

► The interpreter promotes patient autonomy. For example, an interpreter directs a patient who asks him or her for a ride home to appropriate resources within the institution.

CULTURAL AWARENESS

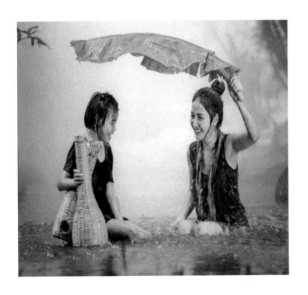

OBJECTIVE: To facilitate communication across cultural differences.

RELATED ETHICAL PRINCIPLE: Interpreters strive to develop awareness of the cultures encountered in the performance of interpreting duties.

► The interpreter strives to understand the cultures associated with the languages he or she interprets, including biomedical culture. For example, an interpreter learns about the traditional remedies some patients may use.

► The interpreter alerts all parties to any significant cultural misunderstanding that arises. For example, if a provider asks a patient who is fasting for religious reasons to take an oral medication, an interpreter may call attention to the potential conflict.

ROLE BOUNDARIES

OBJECTIVE: To clarify the scope and limits of the interpreting role, in order to avoid conflicts of interest.

RELATED ETHICAL PRINCIPLE: The interpreter maintains the boundaries of the professional role, refraining from personal involvement.

► The interpreter limits personal involvement with all parties during the interpreting assignment. For example, an interpreter does not share or elicit overly personal information in conversations with a patient.

► The interpreter limits his or her professional activity to interpreting within an encounter. For example, an interpreter never advises a patient on health care questions, but redirects the patient to ask the provider.

► The interpreter with an additional role adheres to all interpreting standards of practice while interpreting. For example, an interpreter who is also a nurse does not confer with another provider in the patient's presence, without reporting what is said.

PROFESSIONALISM

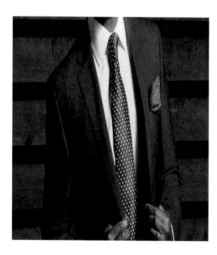

OBJECTIVE: To uphold the public's trust in the interpreting profession.

RELATED ETHICAL PRINCIPLE: Interpreters at all times act in a professional and ethical manner.

► The interpreter is honest and ethical in all business practices. For example, an interpreter accurately represents his or her credentials.

► The interpreter is prepared for all assignments. For example, an interpreter asks about the nature of the assignment and reviews relevant terminology.

► The interpreter discloses skill limitations with respect to particular assignments. For example, an interpreter who is unfamiliar with a highly technical medical term asks for an explanation before continuing to interpret.

► The interpreter avoids sight translation, especially of complex or critical documents, if he or she lacks sight translation skills. For example, when asked to sight translate a surgery consent form, an interpreter instead asks the provider to explain its content and then interprets the explanation.

► The interpreter is accountable for professional performance. For example, an interpreter does not blame others for his or her interpreting errors.

► The interpreter advocates for working conditions that support quality interpreting. For example, an interpreter on a lengthy assignment indicates when fatigue might compromise interpreting accuracy.

► The interpreter shows respect for professionals with whom he or she works. For example, an interpreter does not spread rumors that would discredit another interpreter.

► The interpreter acts in a manner befitting the dignity of the profession and appropriate to the setting. For example, an interpreter dresses appropriately and arrives on time for appointments.

PROFESSIONAL DEVELOPMENT

OBJECTIVE: To attain the highest possible level of competence and service.

RELATED ETHICAL PRINCIPLE: Interpreters strive to further their knowledge and skills, through independent study, continuing education, and actual interpreting practice.

The interpreter continues to develop language and cultural knowledge and interpreting skills.

► For example, an interpreter stays up to date on changes in medical terminology or regional slang.

The interpreter seeks feedback to improve his or her performance.

► For example, an interpreter consults with colleagues about a challenging assignment.

The interpreter supports the professional development of fellow interpreters.

► For example, an experienced interpreter mentors novice interpreters.

The interpreter participates in organizations and activities that contribute to the development of the profession.

► For example, an interpreter attends professional workshops and conferences.

ADVOCACY

OBJECTIVE: To prevent harm to parties that the interpreter serves.

RELATED ETHICAL PRINCIPLE: When the patient's health, well-being or dignity is at risk, an interpreter may be justified in acting as an advocate.

The interpreter may speak out to protect an individual from serious harm.

► For example, an interpreter may intervene on behalf of a patient with a life-threatening allergy, if the condition has been overlooked.

► The interpreter may advocate on behalf of a party or group to correct mistreatment or abuse.

► For example, an interpreter may alert his or her supervisor to patterns of disrespect towards patients.

You can read the entire code of ethics and standards of practice by following the link below: National Standards of Practice for Interpreters in Health Care, https://www.ncihc.org/assets/documents/publications/NCIHC National Standards of Practice.pdf

IMPARTIALITY

A very important basic ethical principle for interpreters is impartiality. Interpreters often work with two parties, and mediate between these parties. A medical interpreter does not work only for the patient or only for the provider, but for both equally. It is important for the interpreter to remember this. Both the provider and the patient need our service. We cannot be focused on only helping one or the other.

Therefore, impartiality means that throughout all communications, the interpreter works to not favor one party over the other party.

WHAT DOES IMPARTIALITY LOOK LIKE?

Impartial interpreters are professionals who must always do the following:

► Refrain from accepting to interpret for family or personal relationships, as it is almost impossible to be impartial to those we care for;

► Remain emotionally detached from the content of the message, as the messages are not ours, even when one of the parties is not the most friendly. The only exception is if discrimination occurs and this will be discussed later on. Withdraw if unable to do so;

► Not judge the content of the messages or any of the parties in the interaction; and

► Ensure that you interpret all the side conversations to both parties so nobody is left out;

► Attempt to analyze who you tend to explain things to more, and realize that you need to balance your interventions and explanations to both parties. Transparency is key to maintain a more impartial stance.

► Remember to always use inclusive language, such as "I am here to interpret for you and the patient", versus "I am here to interpret in Spanish for the patient."

Interpreters must always strive to maintain impartiality. The latest research has ascertained that complete impartiality is impossible and that interpreters are typically more partial to act on behalf of the patient or the provider. It is important for you to always check your behavior and language to minimize this perception. Keep in mind that being impartial does not mean being uncaring. It simply means that you are a mediator who works for two individuals, and in order to do that job well interpreters need to remove themselves from any disagreement or difference of opinion. Working for both parties equally will help enhance the therapeutic rapport. The fact that everyone in healthcare is working for the benefit of the patient may make some interpreters partial to the patient, but just remember that the provider is working for the benefit of the patient too, and any action or behavior should support the provider's effort to do so, versus helping the patient. Impartiality also helps ensure the autonomy of each party.

WHAT DOES PARTIALITY LOOK LIKE?

Any perception that the interpreter prefers the patient over the provider, or vice-versa, will cause the other party to feel like they are at a disadvantage. It erodes the confidence that an individual has on the interpreter, including their expectation that the interpreter will interpret everything without adding, omitting, or changing meaning to help one party over the other. A partial interpreter is seen by others as one who is working for the provider and distancing himself from the patient, or one who identifies very closely with the patient, and therefore, is working primarily for the patient's interests.

PROFESSIONALISM

Interpreters must always act in a professional manner when on an assignment. This includes the following:

► Speaking in a professional tone, using vocabulary that is polite and appropriate for a work environment

► Monitoring one's own performance and behavior to ensure that the interpreter's actions will not interfere with the flow of communication

► Not taking on other roles while you interpret, even if you fulfill other roles in other settings

► Recognizing and stating your limitations in all interactions

► Avoiding potential conflicts of interest and personal involvement

► Not using your position to gain favors from the patient

An interpreter's conduct, behavior, and attitude need to be professional, in order for medical interpreters to be respected by other healthcare professionals. This includes dressing as a professional (or wearing professional attire, such as scrubs where allowed) and having good control over one's emotions. True professionals should consider their appearance, demeanor, reliability, competence, phone and email etiquette, and their professional written correspondence. What one medical interpreter does affects the image of all the other professionals in the field. Affiliation to a professional association, certification, and continuing education are also common expectations of every professional.

RESPECT

Interpreters must respect the autonomy and expertise of all parties in the encounter. If interpreters ever have a question regarding the proper way to show respect to a party, they should consult with the provider or with their agency. Respect does not mean obedience or agreement with something you do not agree with. Respect includes certain qualities, such as always being polite in your language, listening carefully, being helpful and being explicit when one cannot help, and more. It is important that interpreters respect providers and patients equally, regardless of the educational level or other characteristic of either party.

ACCURACY (AND COMPLETENESS)

First, accuracy means that interpreters precisely convey the content and spirit of the message. As an interpreter, you MUST:

► interpret meaning, not words;

► request checks for understanding to ensure the correct message is interpreted;

► intervene to request for clarification (grammatical, semantic, or other), and

► correct any other mistakes that made the interpretation less accurate.

Completeness means not adding any message or omitting any message when interpreting oral or signed language from the source language into the target language. This concept goes hand in hand with accuracy. Completeness is a difficult principle to master because it involves understanding, transforming, and interpreting all the elements of meaning from the source language to the target language.

Faithfulness and fidelity are terms used to describe how close or how faithful the target language is to the source language. Do not confuse fidelity with literal interpretation. A faithful interpretation will elicit the same reaction as if it had been said in the source language, even if with different words.

CONFIDENTIALITY

Interpreters shall not share any assignment-related information with anyone outside the assignment or healthcare team, unless required by law. While sharing issues about certain patients or providers may be tempting, it is highly unethical.

Sometimes, interpreters may describe a case using a limited set of facts and information that does not identify the patient, in order to seek advice from other interpreters or debrief over a difficult case. However, this is for a limited purpose and is one of the only exceptions to the complete confidentiality of the interpreting session.

In addition, interpreters should observe the following requirements of confidentiality:

► Strive to be aware of applicable laws that apply to mandated reporting for abuse or violence;

► Only share experiences for purposes of professional development and only after removing identifying information;

► Clearly explain to both parties that the interpreter will keep everything said confidential at the beginning of interpreting sessions.

ADVOCACY

Interpreters should advocate according to the established procedures of the institution, profession and protocols of their employer or the organization they are working for.

CULTURAL COMPETENCE

Interpreters should continually develop awareness of his or her own culture and other cultures that he or she encounters while interpreting.

10

THE IMIA AND NCHIHC CODES OF ETHICS

LEARNING GOAL

After successful completion of the IMIA and NCIHC Codes of Ethics chapter, participants will be able to do the following:

► Define and apply the IMIA code of ethics and standards of practice for interpreters in the healthcare setting.

LEARNING OBJECTIVES:

Using the above goals, participants should also be able to do the following upon successful completion of this chapter:

► Understand and explain the IMIA code of ethics and standards of practice for interpreters in the healthcare setting.
► Analyze the difference between the IMIA and NCIHC Codes of Ethics.
► Master the IMIA standards of practice and apply them when facing difficult situations or an ethical dilemma.

IMPORTANT TERMS AND WORDS

- ► Maintain confidentiality
- ► Language fluency
- ► Interject personal opinions
- ► Professional judgment
- ► Unobtrusive interventions
- ► Triadic medical setting
- ► Gain favors
- ► Implications
- ► Clinical parameters

- ► Homicidal intent
- ► Child abuse
- ► Domestic violence
- ► Moral fortitude
- ► Conflicts of interest
- ► Scope of employment
- ► Functions or services
- ► Effective strategies

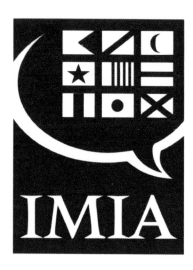

INTERNATIONAL MEDICAL INTERPRETERS ASSOCIATION (IMIA) CODE OF ETHICS

1. Interpreters will maintain confidentiality of all assignment-related information.

2. Interpreters will select the language and mode of interpretation that most accurately conveys the content and spirit of the messages of their clients.

3. Interpreters will refrain from accepting assignments beyond their professional skills, language fluency, or level of training.

4. Interpreters will refrain from accepting an assignment when family or close personal relationships affect impartiality.

5. Interpreters will not interject personal opinions or counsel patients.

6. Interpreters will not engage in interpretations that relate to issues outside the provision of health care services unless qualified to do so.

7. Interpreters will engage in patient advocacy and in the intercultural mediation role of explaining cultural differences/practices to health care providers and patients only when appropriate and necessary for communication purposes, using professional judgment.

8. Interpreters will use skillful unobtrusive interventions so as not to interfere with the flow of communication in a triadic medical setting.

9. Interpreters will keep abreast of their evolving languages and medical terminology.

10. Interpreters will participate in continuing education programs as available.

11. Interpreters will seek to maintain ties with relevant professional organizations in order to be up-to-date with the latest professional standards and protocols.

12. Interpreters will refrain from using their position to gain favors from clients.

IMIA MEDICAL INTERPRETING STANDARDS OF PRACTICE

We would now like to share the section on Ethical Behavior from the Medical Interpreting Standards of Practice that was developed by the International Medical Interpreters Association IMIA & Education Development Center, Inc. The IMIA Healthcare interpreter standards of practice were created to serve as guidelines and very important tools for the interpreters during their interpretation and for their intellectual and professional growth.

EVALUATION METHOD:

The Likert Scale is the rating scale used to evaluate medical interpreting services, with values from 1-5 for which a person will select the number considered to reflect the perceived quality.

LIKERT SCALE

► 5—Fulfills the expectation completely and consistently, with ease and fluidity

► 4—Fulfills the expectation in a mechanical way

► 3—Performs the expectation but with hesitation or lack of confidence

► 2—Performs inconsistently; lapses into behaviors demonstrating lack of mastery

► 1—Is unable to perform the task; exhibits behavior consistent with lack of mastery

DUTY C: ETHICAL BEHAVIOR

C-1 MAINTAIN CONFIDENTIALITY

	INDICATORS OF MASTERY	RATING		INDICATORS OF LACK OF MASTERY
A.	Can explain the boundaries and the meaning of confidentiality, and its implications and consequences	☐ 5 ☐ 4 ☐ 3 ☐ 2 ☐ 1	A.	Cannot explain the boundaries and the meaning of confidentiality, nor its implications and consequences
B.	Knows and maintains the clinical parameters of information sharing, in keeping with the policies and procedures of the institution and/or team, for example: • Supervision • Patient conference / continuity of care meetings • Professional meetings, workshops, conferences, [taking responsibility for maintaining the anonymity of the parties by ensuring that any information shared at professional meetings does not contain identifying characteristics (e.g. hospital names, date of encounter, etc.) that can be attached to a specific individual]	☐ 5 ☐ 4 ☐ 3 ☐ 2 ☐ 1	B.	Intentionally or unintentionally reveals confidential information outside the clinical parameters
C.	Knows how to respond to questions dealing with confidential matters that may be brought up in the community or health care setting	☐ 5 ☐ 4 ☐ 3 ☐ 2 ☐ 1	C.	Does not know how to deflect inappropriate requests for information and violates confidentiality
D.	If privy to information regarding suicidal/ homicidal intent, child abuse, or domestic violence, acts on the obligation to transmit such information in keeping with institutional policies, interpreting standards of practice, the code of ethics, and the law	☐ 5 ☐ 4 ☐ 3 ☐ 2 ☐ 1	D.	Fails to act on the obligation to transmit information to relevant parties

C-2 INTERPRET ACCURATELY AND COMPLETELY

	INDICATORS OF MASTERY	RATING		INDICATORS OF LACK OF MASTERY
A.	Can explain the concepts of accuracy and completeness, and their implications and consequences	☐ 5 ☐ 4 ☐ 3 ☐ 2 ☐ 1	A.	Cannot explain the concept of accuracy and completeness, nor their implications and consequences
B.	Is committed to transmitting accurately and completely the content and spirit of the original message into the other language without omitting, modifying, condensing, or adding	☐ 5 ☐ 4 ☐ 3 ☐ 2 ☐ 1	B.	Is not committed to transmitting accurately and completely the content and spirit of the original message
C.	Is committed to monitoring her or his own interpreting performance	☐ 5 ☐ 4 ☐ 3 ☐ 2 ☐ 1	C.	Does not monitor her or his own interpreting performance
D.	Has the moral fortitude to admit and correct own mistakes	☐ 5 ☐ 4 ☐ 3 ☐ 2 ☐ 1	D.	Does not have the moral fortitude to admit and correct own mistakes, instead permitting mistakes to stand uncorrected

C-3 MAINTAIN IMPARTIALITY

	INDICATORS OF MASTERY	RATING		INDICATORS OF LACK OF MASTERY
A.	Is aware of and able to identify personal biases and beliefs that may interfere with the ability to be impartial, and has the moral fortitude to withdraw if unable to be impartial	☐ 5 ☐ 4 ☐ 3 ☐ 2 ☐ 1	A.	Is unaware of and unable to identify personal biases and beliefs that may interfere with the ability to be impartial, and does not have the moral fortitude to withdraw if unable to be impartial
B.	Withdraws or refrains from accepting any assignment where close personal or professional ties or strong personal beliefs may affect impartiality (including conflicts of interest), unless an emergency renders the service necessary	☐ 5 ☐ 4 ☐ 3 ☐ 2 ☐ 1	B.	Accepts assignments where close personal or professional ties or strong personal beliefs may affect impartiality, even when other alternatives are available

		RATING		
C.	Focuses on the communication between provider and patient and refrains from interjecting personal issues, beliefs, opinions, or biases into the interview	☐ 5 ☐ 4 ☐ 3 ☐ 2 ☐ 1	C.	Interjects personal issues, beliefs, opinions, or biases into the interview
D.	Refrains from counseling or advising	☐ 5 ☐ 4 ☐ 3 ☐ 2 ☐ 1	D.	Counsels and advises

C-4 RESPECT PATIENT'S PRIVACY

	INDICATORS OF MASTERY	RATING		INDICATORS OF LACK OF MASTERY
A.	Respects patient's physical privacy, and maintains spatial/visual privacy of patient, as necessary	☐ 5 ☐ 4 ☐ 3 ☐ 2 ☐ 1	A.	Does not respect patient's physical privacy nor maintain spatial/visual privacy of patient
B.	Respects patient's personal / emotional privacy: • Refrains from asking personal probing questions outside the scope of interpreting tasks • Does not use the role of interpreter to influence a social relationship with the patient outside the interpreting encounter • Refrains from becoming personally involved in the patient's life**	☐ 5 ☐ 4 ☐ 3 ☐ 2 ☐ 1	B.	Does not respect patient's personal/emotional privacy • Asks personal, probing questions on own initiative • Uses the role of interpreter to influence a social relationship with the patient, outside the interpreting encounter • Becomes personally involved

** In small, close-knit communities, it is often not possible for an interpreter to remain personally and socially uninvolved with patients. However, interpreters should always strive to maintain the ethical and professional standards of confidentiality and impartiality while in their role.

C-5 MAINTAIN PROFESSIONAL DISTANCE

	INDICATORS OF MASTERY	RATING		INDICATORS OF LACK OF MASTERY
A.	Can explain the meaning of professional distance, and its implications and consequences	☐5 ☐4 ☐3 ☐2 ☐1	A.	Cannot explain the meaning of professional distance, and its implications and consequences
B.	Is able to balance empathy with the boundaries of the interpreter role	☐5 ☐4 ☐3 ☐2 ☐1	B.	Is not able to balance empathy with the boundaries of the interpreter role
C.	Shows care and concern for patient needs by facilitating the use of appropriate resources	☐5 ☐4 ☐3 ☐2 ☐1	C.	Ignores patient needs or tries to resolve everything for the patient
D.	Refrains from becoming personally involved	☐5 ☐4 ☐3 ☐2 ☐1	D.	Becomes personally involved to the extent of sabotaging or compromising the provider-patient therapeutic relationship, thereby misleading the patient as to who the provider is and effectively disempowering the provider
E.	Does not create expectations in either party that the interpreter role cannot fulfill	☐5 ☐4 ☐3 ☐2 ☐1	E.	Creates expectations in either party that the interpreter role cannot fulfill
F.	Promotes patient self-sufficiency, taking into account the social context of the patient	☐5 ☐4 ☐3 ☐2 ☐1	F.	Encourages and/or creates patient dependency on the interpreter
G.	Monitors own personal agenda and needs and is aware of transference and counter transference issues	☐5 ☐4 ☐3 ☐2 ☐1	G.	Is unaware of transference and counter transference issues

C-6 MAINTAIN PROFESSIONAL INTEGRITY

	INDICATORS OF MASTERY	RATING		INDICATORS OF LACK OF MASTERY
A.	Refrains from contact with the patient outside the scope of employment, avoiding personal benefit	☐ 5 ☐ 4 ☐ 3 ☐ 2 ☐ 1	A.	Initiates contact with the patient outside the scope of employment for personal benefit
B.	Refrains from fulfilling any functions or services that are not part of the interpreter role	☐ 5 ☐ 4 ☐ 3 ☐ 2 ☐ 1	B.	Takes on functions or provides services that are not part of the interpreter role
C.	Knows competency limits and refrains from interpreting beyond her or his training, level of experience, and skills, unless these limitations are fully understood by the patient and provider and no other source of interpreting is available	☐ 5 ☐ 4 ☐ 3 ☐ 2 ☐ 1	C.	Is not aware of competency limits; becomes involved in situations that are beyond her or his level of training, skill, and/or experience; and on occasions where no other source of interpreting is available, does not inform patient or provider of these limitations
D.	Refrains from interpreting in situations where there may be a conflict of interest	☐ 5 ☐ 4 ☐ 3 ☐ 2 ☐ 1	D.	Persists in functioning as an interpreter in situations where there may be a conflict of interest
E.	Engages in ongoing professional development	☐ 5 ☐ 4 ☐ 3 ☐ 2 ☐ 1	E.	Does not engage in ongoing professional development

C-7 DEAL WITH DISCRIMINATION

	INDICATORS OF MASTERY	RATING		INDICATORS OF LACK OF MASTERY
A.	On occasions where the interpreter feels strongly that either party's behavior is affecting access to or quality of service, or compromising either party's dignity, uses effective strategies to address the situation	☐ 5 ☐ 4 ☐ 3 ☐ 2 ☐ 1	A.	Does nothing or addresses the situation in an ineffective, disruptive manner
B.	If the problem persists, knows and uses institutional policies and procedures relevant to discrimination	☐ 5 ☐ 4 ☐ 3 ☐ 2 ☐ 1	B.	Neither knows nor uses institutional policies and procedures relevant to discrimination

To download and read the whole document from the IMIA, please visit: https://imiaweb.org/uploads/pages/102.pdf

For further reading, here are some other important codes of ethics for professional interpreters to apply during their performance:

1. IMIA Guide on Medical Interpreter Ethical Conduct; https://www.imiaweb.org/uploads/pages/380_4.pdf

2. Medical Interpreting Standards of Practice; https://imiaweb.org/uploads/pages/102.pdf

3. California Standards for Healthcare Interpreters Ethical Principles, Protocols, and Guidance on Roles & Intervention; http://www.chiaonline.org/Resources/Documents/CHIA%20Standards/standards_chia.pdf

4. A NATIONAL CODE OF ETHICS FOR INTERPRETERS IN HEALTH CARE; https://www.ncihc.org/assets/documents/publications/NCIHC%20National%20Code%20of%20Ethics.pdf

5. ASTM Standards (Note: Payment may be required to download files); http://www.astm.org/Standards/F2089.htm

6. American Translators Association; https://www.atanet.org/aboutus/index.php

7. Registry for Interpreters for the Deaf; http://www.rid.org/ethics

11

INTERVENTION

LEARNING GOAL

After successful completion of the Intervention chapter, participants will be able to do the following:

► Define and apply the 'The Five Finger Intervention Technique (FFIT)'.

LEARNING OBJECTIVES:

Using the above goals, participants should also be able to do the following upon successful completion of this chapter:

► Understand and know the situations that require intervention.
► Identify the challenges of intervention to be able to follow the Five Finger Intervention Technique effectively.
► Fully understand the importance of transparency during the medical setting.

IMPORTANT TERMS AND WORDS

► Intervention
► Clarification
► A linguistic term
► Non-verbal cues
► Pre-determined phrases
► Glossing over terminology
► Omitting concepts

► Concise
► Transparency
► Transparent communication
► Articulate the message
► Invasive
► Patient-provider therapeutic rapport
► Deflate interpersonal issues

As we mentioned before, the interpreter's goal is to ensure understanding between the patient and the provider. What should the interpreter do if there are other barriers to communication?

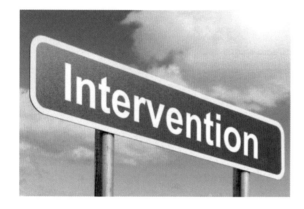

The interpreter may have to take some action or interject with a comment or a question or request for clarification. This is often called intervention, or linguistic or cultural mediation.

In this course, we will refer to the interruptions of the conversation between the provider and the patient to remove barriers as *intervention*.

EXAMPLES OF SITUATIONS NEEDING INTERVENTION

As stated earlier, the interpreter may need to intervene during an interpreting session for many reasons, for example:

A. When the interpreter needs a repetition of what was said,

B. When the interpreter needs to ask the speaker to use shorter phrases,

C. Or when the speaker is not pausing enough to allow for interpretation,

D. When the speaker is looking and talking to the interpreter,

E. When there is a linguistic term that may cause misunderstanding ,

F. Or when there is a cultural concern that may cause misunderstanding, lack of trust, comfort or compliance.

The interpreter will also have to intervene by taking additional steps to clarify the communication. Intervention including clarification may be required when any of the following situations are present:

► The provider or the patient uses complicated or unfamiliar language that the interpreter does not understand;

► The interpreter believes, due to non-verbal cues, that the patient or provider does not understand what is being said;

► A cultural difference presents a barrier to communication between the patient and the provider, etc.

There are many situations where intervention may be required. This requires the interpreter to have well thought out and clear communication strategies, including pre-determined phrases to address common problems.

CHALLENGES OF INTERVENTION

Some interpreters may feel tempted to spend a long time to intervene to "do it the right way" or make everything "just perfect." However, interpreters should only intervene as needed to keep the miscommunication barriers from interfering with the interpreter's ability to interpret and the parties' ability to communicate or focus on the discussion.

In addition to distracting the speaking parties, intervention can be difficult for several reasons. Intervention requires interpreters to come out of the background and speak with their own voice.

This change in positioning and interruption to communication can cause the parties to keep focusing on the interpreter and not each other, even after the barrier to communication has been removed. It is important for the interpreter to indicate when his or her interventions are finished and to give the parties instructions to resume, if necessary. Providers are professionals in a position of authority. Intervening requires a good deal of self-confidence and professional competence from the interpreter.

However, there are also negative consequences to not intervening. A perfect flow of communication is not a mark of a flawless interpretation. Not requesting a clarification when needed may ultimately mean the interpreter is glossing over terminology, adding or omitting concepts inadvertently, due to not addressing the demands of the situation.

Ineffective intervention can cause a breakdown in the relationship between the patient and the provider as well as undermine the students' trust in the interpreter. Therefore, an interpreter needs to be able to intervene effectively and this will be practiced in the medical practice sessions.

THE FIVE FINGER INTERVENTION TECHNIQUE (FFIT)

How does the interpreter intervene? Interpreters can use the Five Finger Intervention Technique when they need to intervene to ensure effective communication among all parties. Here are the steps to follow the Five Finger Intervention Technique (FFIT):

1. The interpreter should raise their hand or change their positioning to signal non-verbally to the parties that they are going to interrupt the conversation. If this is not possible (as in OPI or VRI), they will do it verbally, as described below. The interpreter should already mention and explain the signal of raising their hand when they introduce themselves to both parties before the session starts.

2. The interpreter should use the **third person** (e.g. "The interpreter requests..." or "this is the interpreter speaking") so that the parties are not confused and they know that the interpreter is currently speaking on behalf of him or herself.

3. The interpreter should be clear, concise, and brief, and not spend a lot of time when they intervene. The interpreter should limit the intervention to only one question or to one or two comments (e.g. "There is a lot of noise in the hallway, the interpreter would like to close the door"). It can be helpful to have 'ready-to-use' phrases prepared in advance for the most common situations.

4. The interpreter should always be transparent and tell the other party what he/she tells the first party. This means saying the same message twice, once in each language. This ensures that trust in the interpreter is maintained. The interpreter must always be transparent with any side dialogues that occur.

5. The interpreter should alert the parties when to resume, then go back to the conduit role and start interpreting in the first person again.

THE IMPORTANCE OF TRANSPARENCY

TRANSPARENT COMMUNICATION simply means that each party always knows what the interpreter and the other party have said or signed. For example, if the provider uses a term that has no linguistic equivalent in the target language, the interpreter should let the provider know that they will need to explain this term when interpreting to the patient. This way, the provider understands why the interpreter is asking the patient a question or taking a much longer time to articulate the message than it took to say in the source language.

ADDITIONAL RECOMMENDATIONS

► A good problem-solving intervention should be quick, smooth, and effective in either resolving a problem or bringing it to the provider's or patient's attention. Following these guidelines can help the interpreter to intervene more smoothly and effectively during the medical interpreting appointment.

► The interpreter should not feel uncomfortable or even emotional when they intervene for clear communication among all the parties. If patients see that the interpreter is troubled, they could also become worried or emotional. Therefore, interpreters should always have self-confidence when intervening.

► Interpreters should not assume that they know what the patient is thinking or feeling. If interpreters suspect there is a problem (including confusion or a pressing concern), the interpreter should bring that to the attention of all parties by intervening instead of assuming that the patient or the provider does not understand or does not care.

► The interpreter should go back to the conduit role after they finish the intervention. The provider and the patient will be able to resolve the problem.

► Sometimes an interpreter's intervention may solve the problem directly; for example, by asking for a clarification of a term. Other times, the intervention shows the party that the problem may exist, and the provider or the patient must take the next step. For example, when an interpreter asks a patient if he/she understands, and he/she says "no," it is best to simply interpret the response and let the provider decide to handle the situation.

Intervening too often or too aggressively can cause problems. The more invasive a role the interpreter takes, the greater the risk of getting in the way of the patient-provider relationship. However, if an interpreter takes a role that is too limited, and doesn't intervene as necessary, misunderstandings may also occur that undermine the critical patient-provider therapeutic rapport or the patient's health. Intervention is therefore a difficult task that should be approached incrementally (*i.e.* in increasing steps).

MORE EXAMPLES OF INTERVENTION TECHNIQUES

As we mentioned before, interpreters may need to interject when a message is continuing for too long or remind a party to slow down during the interpreting session. In face-to-face encounters when necessary, interpreters should begin problem solving by raising their hand, standing, or even moving between the provider and the patient if appropriate. In OPI and VRI, verbal indicators are necessary, and usually started with "Excuse me. The interpreter..."

Then, interpreters should remember to state what was just said to the other party and go back to resume interpreting.

These interventions take more confidence and care than common problem solving.

There are other intervention techniques that involve intercultural mediation, patient advocacy and de-escalation techniques, which medical interpreters learn in hospitals, or that involve helping deflate interpersonal issues that may arise, which we will discuss later.

12

INCREMENTAL INTERVENTION

LEARNING GOAL

After successful completion of the Incremental Intervention chapter, participants will be able to do the following:

► Define the concept of Incremental Intervention and apply it effectively when they have to intervene while in a medical interpreting setting.

LEARNING OBJECTIVES:

Using the above goals, participants should also be able to do the following upon successful completion of this chapter:

► Understand and explain the concept of incremental intervention to be able to intervene effectively during a medical interpreting setting.
► Give more examples of incremental intervention.
► Explain when the interpreter should shift to simultaneous mode of interpreting.

IMPORTANT TERMS AND WORDS

► Incremental intervention
► Invasive intervention

► Significant

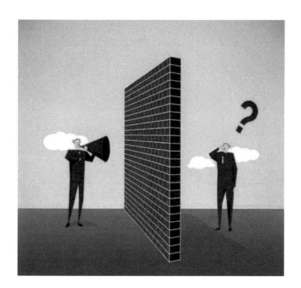

(This concept was originated by Cynthia E. Roat and is the basis of the CCHCP's "Bridging the Gap" interpreter training model.)

INCREMENTAL INTERVENTION happens when interpreters start with the least invasive intervention that might solve the problem and move incrementally towards more invasive, or assertive, interventions to remove a communication barrier. If that intervention does not produce the desired effect (i.e. asking a patient to look at the provider), the intervention or request may have to be repeated. If the second intervention does not work, the interpreter may have other options, such as change positioning to help the patient look at the provider. If the communicative barrier is significant and the interpreter cannot play their role effectively, the interpreter has the option to request to be replaced. The replaced interpreter should intervene as needed to ensure effective communication, and resume interpreting after finishing the intervention.

MORE EXAMPLES OF INCREMENTAL INTERPRETING

First, imagine a situation where a provider insists on speaking for many sentences before pausing for interpretation, and the interpreter can only remember two to three sentences at a time. In this situation, the interpreter appropriately raises her hand and speaks as the interpreter to request that the provider speak in short and simple phrases.

However, the provider soon ignores or forgets the problem-solving request and goes back to speaking for long periods. The interpreter then steps into the conduit role again, and this time he/she also requests that the provider remember that the interpreter has a limited memory to be able to accurately interpret what the provider says.

This second intervention is more assertive than the first, because it includes a reason the interpreter needs to solve the problem. The reason should always be patient safety focused, so the provider can relate to and appreciate the medical repercussions of meaningful and accurate communication in healthcare. However, the provider soon forgets again and continues to speak in longer and longer segments.

> The interpreter should shift to simultaneous mode of interpreting or start taking notes to be able to remember everything that is said.

In a second example, the interpreter is in a session where a social worker is trying to understand where a child was left alone when an accident occurred. The patient, who speaks Spanish, explains that the child was in the "solar" at the time. The provider speaks some Spanish, and she assumes that the word "solar" in Spanish means a sunroom and is inside the house.

Further questions by the provider about where the "solar" is in the house, only confuses the patient. Sensing a breakdown in communication, the interpreter raises her hand to problem solve.

Here, the interpreter could adopt the role of cultural mediator to explain that in Honduras many people refer to the area around their home such as a porch or patio as being "in" or "at" their home. However, the interpreter decides to ask the provider to clarify with the LEP person what she means by the word "solar." After the provider asks the patient what a "solar" is, the patient explains that she is talking about the yard, and the miscommunication is solved.

13

PROBLEM SOLVING

LEARNING GOAL

After successful completion of the Problem-Solving chapter, participants will be able to do the following:

► Define and explain how to solve a problem during the medical interpreting setting.

LEARNING OBJECTIVES:

Using the above goals, participants should also be able to do the following upon successful completion of this chapter:

► Understand and explain the concept of solving a problem; and be able to solve the problems one may face during a medical interpreting setting effectively.

► Give more examples of the challenging problems that the interpreters might face during the medical interpreting encounter, and how they should attempt to solve them effectively.

► Realize that some problems do not require intervention (and be able to give examples for these problems).

► Identify the different relationships in an interpreting session.

IMPORTANT TERMS AND WORDS

► Problem of ambiguity
► Good judgment

► Scope of practice
► Therapeutic rapport

Problem Solving Quotes

No problem can be solved from the same level of consciousness that created it

Albert Einstein

So far, we have discussed intervention and explained when the interpreters should intervene and how they should follow the Five Finger Intervention Technique to manage linguistic, cultural, and other types of barriers.

Problem solving is undoubtedly part of the act of interpreting. If you need to ask for clarification, you are attempting to solve a problem of ambiguity. Some people may seem to think that interpreting is just the rendering, and that problem solving is separate. However, the truth is that problem solving is tightly embedded in the act of interpreting, which is why it is now being seen more as a mediation practice, and not a linguistic practice alone.

In this section, we will discuss different kinds of problems that can be solved by interpreters without intervening. There is indeed a difference between intervention and problem solving.

Problem solving examples that do not require intervention include:

- ▶ asking someone to close the door due to undue noise;

- ▶ moving to the other side to hear better;

- ▶ explaining a role when there is confusion; and

- ▶ doing a debrief to prevent a problem.

- ▶ The following includes other examples of problems that interpreters may face and how they should attempt to solve the problem based on the situation:

- ▶ The provider asks the interpreter to sight translate a long or complicated document. The interpreter should refuse politely and mention the reason for his refusal and recommend any solutions that may be available.

- ▶ The provider asks the interpreter to translate a document for a patient, but it is not part of the interpreter's job to translate. The interpreter should politely refuse to translate the document and tell the provider that he/she is an interpreter not a certified translator, explaining that there is a big difference between translation and interpretation and both of them require different sets of skills. The interpreter should also remind the provider of liability in case he/she makes a mistake in translating this document.

► The patient might offer a gift to the interpreter. The interpreter should refuse politely saying that he/she cannot accept any gifts and it is the policy of the employer.

► The patient might ask the interpreter to babysit her kids while the patient is busy doing something. The interpreter should tell the patient that this is not a part of the scope of the practice and that he or she cannot do that.

There are many other problems that will require the interpreter to use good judgment and fully understand the scope of practice for professional interpreters. This means being aware of what they should or should not do and which activities are parts of their jobs and which are not. In cases when they cannot solve a problem on their own, interpreters should feel comfortable seeking the advice of their supervisors or colleagues.

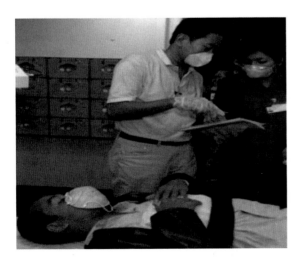

THE RELATIONSHIPS IN THE INTERPRETING SESSION

There are at least three relationships in any interpreting session:

1. The relationship between the patient and the provider;

2. The relationship between the patient and the interpreter; and

3. The relationship between the provider and the interpreter.

Out of the three relationships above, the patient and provider relationship is the most important, and is called the *therapeutic rapport*. To understand why it is the most important, studies tell us to imagine that both the provider and the patient speak the same language. In this case, the patient-interpreter and the provider-interpreter relationships would be unnecessary because the patient and the provider would directly communicate with one another without the interpreter.

However, when there are two different languages being used, an interpreter will have to step in to enable communication between provider and patient. This makes the interpreter instrumental for the development of the primary therapeutic relationship, and therefore, must take care to support and not undermine that relationship. As stated in the IMIA Standards of Practice, the interpreter "manages the flow of communication to enhance the patient-provider relationship (IMIA A-11: A)."

14

ENSURING UNDERSTANDING

LEARNING GOAL

► After successful completion of the Ensuring Understanding chapter, participants will be able to ensure understanding of the listener and to check understanding.

LEARNING OBJECTIVES:

Using the above goals, participants should also be able to do the following upon successful completion of this chapter:

► Understand the main responsibility of the interpreter.
► Realize the importance of checking understanding.
► Explain the term 'teach back' and when it is necessary to use.

IMPORTANT TERMS AND WORDS

► Teach back
► Non-verbal cues
► Puzzled expression
► Distracted eye contact

The interpreter should be aware of non-verbal cues that indicate a lack of understanding such as a puzzled expression or distracted eye contact. These are prompts to check for understanding. According to the IMIA Standards of Practice, it is the interpreter's responsibility to "ensure that the listener understands the message" (IMIA A-8). This means ensuring the understanding of all parties, including the interpreter.

If interpreters suspect that someone is confused, they should intervene. They might say to the provider, "the interpreter would like to ensure that the patient has understood." The provider now knows that the interpreter wants to check to see if the patient needs clarification, and the provider can decide what to do next.

An important task for practicing medical interpreters is to invite providers to do what is referred to as "teach back". In the past, a check for understanding was normally practiced. A check for understanding happens when a provider asks the patient if he or she understands, and the answer is usually yes, whether the patient understands or not. Evidently, asking someone if they understood is not a very useful tactic as many people will be afraid to say they do not. As a result, **Teach Back** is now encouraged in healthcare. This is when the provider asks the patient to explain what he or she understands about what was just explained. This forces the patient to rephrase the concept as understood as a way for the provider to ascertain if the patient adequately understands the concept.

> Sometimes the provider may ask the interpreter to do teach back directly with the patient and relay the patient's answer. In other cases, the provider may decide to do nothing at all. In these instances, interpreters should not insist but should remain professional and neutral unless the patient's safety, life, health, or dignity is at risk.

NOTES

15

REGISTER

LEARNING GOAL

► After successful completion of the Register chapter, participants will be able to understand the term register and its relationship with delivering accurate and complete message.

LEARNING OBJECTIVES:

Using the above goals, participants should also be able to do the following upon successful completion of this chapter:

► Understand the main concept of register and "five-term distinction".
► Give examples of the differences between high-register and low-register speech.
► Explain how and when the interpreter can lower the register.

IMPORTANT TERMS AND WORDS

► Register
► Five-term distinction
► Linguistic varieties

► Formality
► Fundamental idea
► Amputate

Quirk et. al. (1989, 25) present a "five-term distinction" to categorize linguistic varieties, and they narrow down the range of registers to:

Very Formal–FORMAL–Neutral– INFORMAL–Very Informal

The very formal variety of language ("extremely distant, rigid or frozen"; Quirk et. al. 1989, 27) is often found in written instructions. Very informal language, which is also called 'intimate, casual, slangy, or hearty' (ibid.) is used between family members or close friends. Knowing this scale can be very useful for interpreters when trying to assess the party's register level.

Source: http://www.glottopedia.org/index. php/Register_(discourse)

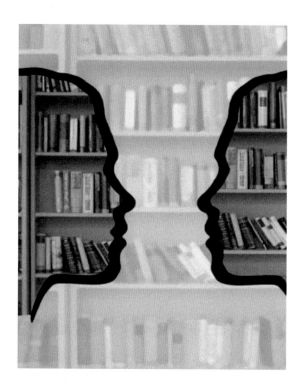

REGISTER means the level of formality or complexity of the language a person or professional uses. High register speech is very formal and complex. The professional and skilled interpreter may have the ability to lower the register of speech which means to take something that was said in a very formal, complex way and say it in a simpler and easier to understand way based on the literacy level of the listener.

If the interpreter decides to lower the register, he or she should consider the following:

1. Duration of the message; when interpreting into the lower register, the interpreter must maintain a similar duration as the high register message

2. The fundamental idea/meaning should be the same

3. The interpreter should not explain. Lowering the register does not mean explaining–explaination is the job of the provider.

Register is also a key part of communicative accuracy. Register, in a general sense, means the language which is used by professionals who share the same profession. For example, teachers, doctors, interpreters, lawyers and other professionals use a certain register when they speak.

Generally, medical interpreters should not change the register of the speech they interpret for, based on traditional interpreting practices. However, medical interpreting requires ensuring understanding. So, if a patient does not understand a provider's speech because of the high register and the provider does not try to lower the register to help the patient fully understand everything he/she needs to know, the interpreter's best course of action is to intervene and directly ask the provider to ensure understanding or lower the register. In medical interpreting, it is acceptable to lower the provider's register when the interpreter is confident of the meaning and other incremental interventions have not worked. Interpreters should pay extra attention to high register when working with survivors of trauma. Interpreters should never increase the register of a response to make a speaker or speech sound better.

Below are a few examples of the differences between high-register and low-register speech:

- ► High register: Your pains were acute.

- ► Low register: Your pains were quick to become bad.

- ► High register: We had to amputate your son's leg.

- ► Low register: We had to permanently remove your son's leg surgically.

16

MANAGING THE FLOW OF THE SESSION

LEARNING GOAL

► After successful completion of the Managing the Flow of the Session chapter, participants will be able to understand how to manage the session effectively.

LEARNING OBJECTIVES:

Using the above goals, participants should also be able to do the following upon successful completion of this chapter:

► Manage the flow of the session professionally and effectively.

► Understand the first-person and how to use the first-person.

► Explain the differences between the usage of first-person and third-person.

► Realize when to switch from the first person to the third person.

► Know to position yourself in the medical setting and why positioning is important.

► Explain the importance of pre-session and know to deliver an effective pre-session with the patient and the provider.

► Avoid side conversation.

IMPORTANT TERMS AND WORDS

- ► Transparent exchange
- ► Facilitation
- ► First person
- ► Reported speech
- ► Culturally inappropriate
- ► Physical position
- ► Positioning

- ► Billing conversations
- ► Scheduling appointments
- ► A phrase-by-phrase
- ► Subject Matter
- ► 3x5 rule
- ► Side Conversations

B y now, you should understand the basic steps of intervention and the complexity of the interpreter's roles. Next, we will address managing the flow of the session and performing the role of cultural mediator.

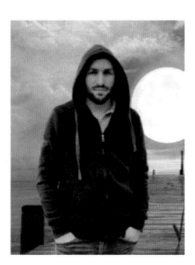

Interpreters are in charge of making sure that there is a transparent exchange of meaning between the parties during the interpreting session because interpreters are often the only professionals in the room that understand both sides of the

conversation equally well. In other words, interpreters are in charge of making sure that the parties speak in a way that can be accurately and completely interpreted. This requires some facilitation skills. In communication, the term facilitation or facilitator refers to enabling a group to communicate effectively. (IMIA, A-10).

THE FIRST PERSON AND WHY WE SHOULD USE THE FIRST PERSON

Interpreters usually work in the "first person" when they interpret. **First person** speech means that interpreters interpret for the individual without changing any pronouns, speaking *as* the individual.

For example, if a social worker says, "may I come in?" the interpreter should interpret "may I come in?" and not "she asks if she can come in" or even "may we come in."

This form of speaking, referred to as first person speech, is more efficient and clearer once the parties understand the interpreter's role. When interpreters do not use first person to interpret what others are saying (*e.g.* she says...), interpreters refer to the interpretation as **reported speech**.

In addition to being shorter and clearer, the use of first person is better than the use of reported speech because it:

► Helps to strengthen the primary relationship between the provider and patient;

► Helps the patient and provider speak directly to each other;

► Helps the interpreter to stay in the background, and not be the focus of attention; and

► Helps the interpreter to focus on interpreting exactly what was said.

(adapted from the 2014 Bridging the Gap: Medical Interpreter Training presentation by Cross Cultural Health Care Program)

Many new interpreters and sometimes end users of the service find first person speech uncomfortable at first, but with practice it becomes more natural.

There is an exception to this rule. The IMIA Standard recognizes that sometimes the third person is needed, as it states that the interpreter "Uses the first person ("I") form as the standard, but can switch to the third person, when the first-person form or direct speech causes confusion *or is culturally inappropriate* (IMIA Standards A-7). This may include a situation with a young child or a mental health patient who may be confused as to who is speaking, for example.

POSITIONING IN MEDICAL INTERPRETING

The interpreter's physical position within a room can have a large influence on how the patient and the provider relate to one another. It also affects the interpreter's ability to listen to all speakers. In interpreting, we refer to **positioning** as the physical location of the provider, the patient, and the interpreter.

Interpreters should strive to position themselves in a way that facilitates and encourages communication between the patient and the provider. The interpreter should be unobtrusive (*i.e.* not in the way), and direct eye contact between the patient and the provider should be encouraged through the interpreter's **positioning and gaze** (*i.e.* who the interpreter looks at).

Ideally, interpreters will select a position next to or slightly behind the patient or provider. This depends on many variables, and will be further discussed in the practice sessions. It may not always be possible for the interpreter to be in his or her ideal position, but interpreters should try to consider several factors:

► The ability to hear all parties to be interpreted

► Encouragement of direct patient-provider eye gaze

► Position that doesn't require too much neck turning back and forth

► Position that ensures interpreter safety in certain cases.

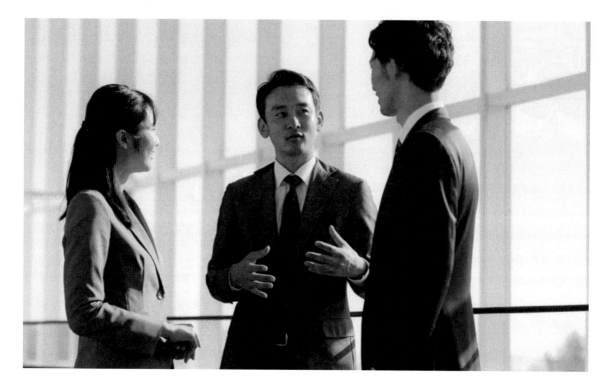

Sometimes, it is uncomfortable for a patient to have the interpreter behind them because they have less experience with the interpreter.

Sometimes, standing next to the provider gives the patient more autonomy as well.

Last, even though the triangle scenario is not encouraged typically, it can work in some instances. For in-patient scenarios, the interpreter sometimes needs to be on the other side of the bed or in between the provider and patient in order to hear the bedridden patient.

HOW TO POSITION ONESELF

There are many situations where the ideal position for the interpreter may not be clear. For instance, there may be many patient family members present (sitting to the side of the family members may be an option), or the parties may be moving from place to place as the interpreter interprets (staying close enough to hear is the most important factor here). There also may not be any room to sit or stand beside the provider or patient. In this case, it may be necessary to explain that one needs to change positioning.

> Remember, we can't ask to do our job, we need to do it. Interpreters are not technicians, they are practice professionals.

Because each situation is different, interpreters need to actively decide where it is most appropriate to sit or stand to best ensure that the parties communicate directly with one another and do not address the interpreter. Direct communication is more efficient and contributes to a more equal power balance between the patient and the provider.

SOME COMMON TYPES OF INTERACTIONS INTERPRETERS ENCOUNTER

Interpreting can take place during a dialogue (i.e. a back-and-forth conversation), a question-and-answer session, or a speech, among other formats. There are often only two speakers, in addition to the interpreter, but there may be more participants to the communicative event, such as a spouse, family members, or other relatives.

The consecutive mode of interpreting is used in most medical interpreting encounters because it is the easiest for parties to understand and the simplest for interpreters to use, as it requires no equipment. These include patient interviews, billing conversations, scheduling appointments, patient examinations, and many other encounters. Interpreters will switch out of consecutive mode if there is a need to do so, such as when a patient needs emergency care and will not pause for the interpreter.

Each of the above situations has specific characteristics and needs for which interpreters must be thoroughly prepared. These settings may be interpreted in person or over the telephone. Medical interpreting is most often performed on a phrase-by-phrase basis, with rapid alternation between the speaker and interpreter. Occasionally, however, longer questions or answers may require that the interpreter take notes and retain long passages of messages to avoid disrupting the flow of communication.

Telephonic interpreting poses a challenge to the interpreter because of the lack of visual cues, such as gestures and facial expressions, which provide vital information that the interpreter can use to clarify meaning or intent. To make up for the lack of visual input, the interpreter may need to intervene more frequently to interpret short phrases or to request repetitions or clarifications. In some cases, facilities are equipped with video connections that can make up for this shortcoming, but that is not always possible.

Even with a video connection, remote interpreting still presents a different set of challenges compared to in-person interpreting, due to lack of complete visual cues and possible variable noise distractions. Background noise that would not be as much of a distraction in an in-person setting can be extremely disturbing to an interpreter working with a telephone or video connection. That is why in all remote interpreting cases, it is important to ensure a good audio connection with limited auditory interference.

SUBJECT MATTER TOO COMPLEX FOR THE INTERPRETER

Some interpreting assignments are more complex than others. For example, medical studies may require very specialized and even rare condition discussions and require assignment preparation. Whenever a specialty is unfamiliar to the interpreter, the interpreter should consider whether to refuse or withdraw from the assignment. If an interpreter believes she may be able to accept the assignment but is not sure, the interpreter can use **the 3x5 rule**, meaning that if the interpreter needs to look up more than three unfamiliar terms or ask for explanation more than three times in the first five minutes, and the medical terminology is beyond the interpreter's linguistic skills, the interpreter should consider withdrawal from the assignment (explained in more detail in the coming sections). All of us have our limits and you must know your abilities and your limits to decide the best action to take in certain situations. Disclosing a lack of familiarity with certain highly technical terminology is a sign of professionalism and not of incompetency.

SPEAKING WITH THE PARTIES OUTSIDE THE SESSION

Many patients and providers have limited experience with working with interpreters. It is important to educate both the patient and the provider how to work successfully with an interpreter through the **pre-session**.

Communications with providers outside of the interpreting session are often simple emails or phone calls to arrange the time, date, and place of interpretation, but they

may also involve a quick discussion of the interpreter's role, introductions, and the subject of interpretation.

Whenever these preliminary conversations occur before an interpreting assignment and involve more than just a simple arrangement of the interpreting session, interpreters refer to this conversation as the **pre-session**.

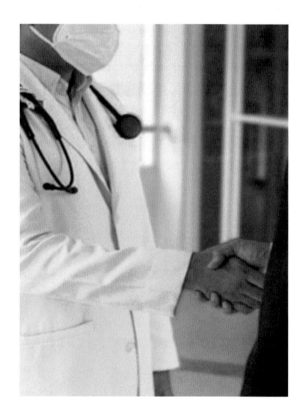

PRE-SESSION

Pre-session can help the interpreters to solve several potential problems and challenges that might cause a lot of headaches for both the interpreter and the parties. Pre-sessions commonly occur before the interpreting session begins, but they can occur at any time prior to the session, with the provider and/or patient.

A pre-session is the best opportunity to avoid problems before they arise. Interpreters can use this time to explain the purpose of their role and strategies that interpreters use, and to ask any questions before the interpreting begins.

A pre-session not only helps build a professional rapport and trust between interpreters and providers or patients, but also provides interpreters with an opportunity to explain how the interpretation will work.

Some examples of what to do in a pre-session with the provider, include the following:

- Greeting (good morning, hello…);
- The interpreter's full name and company;
- Mention the language / dialect that you speak;
- Describe the interpreter's role. For example: "I will ensure accurate and complete communication between x and y, by interpreting everything that is said in confidence";
- Request that the provider speak directly to the patient, not to the interpreter;
- Explain that the interpreter will interpret everything that is said during the interpreting session, not just what the provider wants the interpreter to say;

- Explain that the interpreter may need clarification to do so;
- Explain that interpreters sometimes take notes and that the notes will be destroyed;
- Explain that the interpreting session will be kept confidential;
- Explain that the interpreter will need to position himself/herself for effective interpretation;
- Ask if the provider will need any document to be sight translated;
- Explain the use of first person instead of indirect speech;

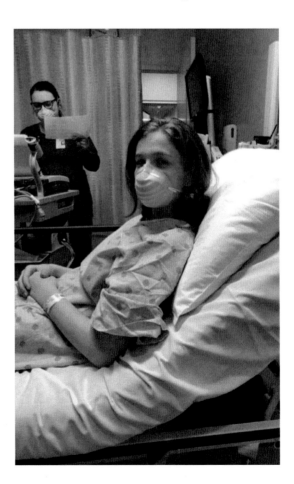

Ask the provider to speak in very short sentences as much as possible for accurate interpretation;

► Answer any appropriate questions from the provider;

► Ask the provider if there is anything special about this session that you should know before you start. When possible, hold a pre-conference to find out the provider's goals for the encounter and other relevant background information. (Adapted from: A-1 IMIA Standards of practice).

AVOID SIDE CONVERSATIONS

When interpreters exchange a conversation with the patient, family member, or providers but do not interpret it during an interpreting session, this is called a **side conversation**. Side conversations cannot always be avoided, but they make the interpreter responsible for relaying the information later, which one may forget to do. This is why interpreters should always be careful to make sure everything they discuss separately with one party is also interpreted afterward to the other party. *Never have a side conversation with a patient without being transparent and interpreting what was said to the provider.*

NOTES

17

ACTIVE LISTENING & MEMORY DEVELOPMENT

LEARNING GOAL

- After successful completion of the Active Listening and Memory Development chapter, participants will be able to listen actively and understand the concept of memory development.

LEARNING OBJECTIVES:

Using the above goals, participants should also be able to do the following upon successful completion of this chapter:

- Fully understand the concept of active listening.
- Know the difference between hearing and listening.
- Explain the different strategies to improve active listening skills.
- Know and illustrate the three types of memory.
- Know the short-term and long-term memory enhancement techniques and how to apply them to enhance their memory.

IMPORTANT TERMS AND WORDS

- Active listening
- Memory development
- Crucial
- SOLER
- Parroting

- Fundamental idea
- Take Notes
- Visualization
- Word association

In this section, we will talk about one of the most important soft skills that professional interpreters must develop and practice—active listening. Additionally, we will discuss memory development and some techniques for how interpreters can better retain information.

DIFFERENCE BETWEEN HEARING AND LISTENING

According to Merriam-Webster Dictionary, the definition of **hearing** is the process, function, or power of perceiving sound. Meanwhile, the definition of **listening** is to hear something with thoughtful attention: give consideration.

Hearing is passive because it happens involuntarily. You can hear what other people around you are saying but it is your choice to focus on what is being said or not. On the other hand, listening is an active process whereby we consciously make the effort to pay attention and fully understand the speaker's speech.

ACTIVE LISTENING

The National Council on Interpreting in Health Care defines the term active listening as the following: "A skill or method of listening that focuses on what is being said for content and purpose in order to achieve full understanding."

Since interpreters must convey the exact message and intent of the original speaker, genuine active listening is crucial to the effectiveness of an interpreter. Active listening is one of the best skills that medical interpreters can benefit from since it will allow them to better understand all parties and deliver more accurate and complete interpretation. To develop your active listening skill, you must consciously listen to everything is said. You must pay attention and not be distracted by anything around you or lose focus or concentration on the speaker's message.

A great technique that teaches interpreters how to actively listen is SOLER. Gerard Egan (1986) in his book "The Skilled Helper" created this acronym SOLER which stands for:

S: Sit SQUARELY,

O: Maintain an OPEN posture,

L: LEAN slightly in towards the client,

E: Maintain EYE CONTACT with the client without staring, and

R: RELAX.

STRATEGIES TO IMPROVE ACTIVE LISTENING SKILLS

Below is a list of strategies to practice and follow regularly to improve your active listening skills:

CONCENTRATE AND PAY FULL ATTENTION

► Look at the speaker and have eye contact if it is appropriate.

► Do not get distracted by anything around you such as another conversation nearby, background activity and noise, or your thoughts, feelings, or biases. Remind yourself to focus and pay attention again when your mind drifts.

► Pay attention to your body language and show respect to the speaker regardless of what he/she is saying.

► Listen without Judgement

► Listen and fully understand the speaker's message regardless of what you think about the speaker (if they are honest or dishonest, good or bad).

► Be neutral and do not criticize, judge, or make assumptions about the speaker.

PARROTING

► Also called oral repetition, parroting is repeating verbatim (word for word) what the speaker says, in the same language. This exercise can help you practice active listening, but be careful that you still remember the meaning of the message rather than just the words used.

MAIN (FUNDAMENTAL) IDEA

► When listening, identify the main idea and the meaning of what is said instead of focusing on memorizing every word.

► Remember that a verbatim rendition is not accurate because every language has its own syntax and grammatical structure.

ASK FOR CLARIFICATION

► Don't be afraid to play your role as a clarifier if you need to clear any misunderstanding or if there is a barrier to understanding the message.

TAKE NOTES

► Take effective notes to remember what is said if the speaker goes on and on and he/she does not want to stop. (Note-taking will be discussed in the next section).

Mastering the active listening skill will require consistent practice. Keep training your mind to concentrate on what the speaker is saying and avoid getting distracted by other thoughts or your surroundings. By being an active listener, you can become more successful in your medical interpreting assignments and provide better communication between the provider and patient.

THE THREE TYPES OF MEMORY

Memories are all created in the brain, but your brain remembers some things longer or better than others because of how well the information is stored. Generally speaking, there are three types of memory storage that the brain uses: Sensory

Memory, Short-Term Memory, and Long-Term Memory.

Sensory Memory is the brain's ability to remember most things you saw or heard within the last five to seven seconds, even if you were not paying close attention. For example, if someone calls your name and you realize that they asked you a question, you may be able to recall the question exactly even if you were not actively listening.

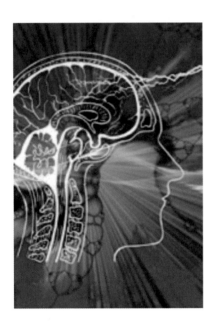

Sensory Memory is useful for interpreting short exchanges. Usually, these rapid-fire exchanges do not require notes because your brain is able to retain this information through Sensory Memory.

Second, **Short-Term Memory** is used for things you saw, heard, or experienced in any span of time longer than about seven seconds but no longer than a day or two ago. Memory enhancement techniques for interpreters mostly focus on this type of

memory storage because longer consecutive interpreting can overwhelm the brain's Short-Term Memory storage abilities.

Lastly, **Long-Term Memory** storage is used for retaining information beyond a day or two. This is the most permanent of memory storage types. However, much of what we experience does not become Short-Term Memory, and much of our Short-Term Memory does not become Long-Term Memory. An example of Long-Term Memory for interpreters is the ability to remember symbols and abbreviations that you create to aid you in your note-taking.

SHORT-TERM MEMORY ENHANCEMENT TECHNIQUES

There are several techniques you can use to improve your short-term memory when interpreting; however, these techniques will not give you superpowers. Always keep in mind that your short-term memory worsens as you get tired or distracted by physical discomfort, thirst, hunger, noises, or the need to use the restroom.

15125551212

1 (512) 555 1212

First, **chunking** means organizing information into groups that are easier to remember. For example, instead of remembering the number 574,833 you could remember 57-48-33. Mentally sorting the information into smaller, organized "chunks" will assist you, and you can organize and label these chunks of information in any way that you will remember them. With chunking, any association that you can make to simplify the information works!

Second, **visualization** is when the interpreter imagines a picture or scenario. Many interpreters imagine that they are experiencing what an LEP person describes when they are relating their medical history or condition. Visualization is a great technique because it encourages active listening and can help interpreters remember even detailed descriptions and directions.

Interpreters can visualize a message even when the content is not obviously visual. Some interpreters report imagining labels on objects with descriptions or using concept maps to visualize a process. Visualization is an individual process, and anything descriptive or even silly that you devise will be a helpful memory aid.

Lastly, **word association** can help you increase your short-term memory by linking a word with a concept you are already familiar with. Word association can help with remembering long lists by associating the sound, spelling, or personal associations the interpreter already has with a word. For example, an interpreter could remember the names of several family members by associating each family member with a piece of fruit that starts with the same letter: A family with five members (Anne, Josh, Gary, Mary, and Terry) could become five fruits (apple, jalapeno, guava, mango, and tomatoes) and their ages could be written on the fruit.

In general, experienced interpreters have their limits both regarding the length of a message they can remember and how long they can interpret. While an interpreter's message length limit varies greatly from interpreter to interpreter, a good rule to follow for how long to interpret is the "rule of two and twenty"—don't interpret for more than two hours at a time in consecutive or twenty minutes at a time in simultaneous.

LONG-TERM MEMORY ENHANCEMENT TECHNIQUES

Just as cramming for a test is not the most effective way to remember something long-term, trying to learn many new symbols in a single, long practice session is not the most effective technique.

> To increase your long-term memory retention of symbols and abbreviations, try practicing at different times of day, in different places, and over many occasions.

18

BASIC NOTE-TAKING FOR INTERPRETERS

LEARNING GOAL

► After successful completion of the Basic Note-Taking for Interpreters chapter, participants will be able to know the basics of taking notes during the interpreting encounter.

LEARNING OBJECTIVES:

Using the above goals, participants should also be able to do the following upon successful completion of this chapter:

► Fully understand the basics of taking notes during their medical interpreting encounter.
► Explain how to practice taking notes.
► Know what they should avoid while taking notes.

IMPORTANT TERMS AND WORDS

► Distractor   ► Symbols and abbreviations

Interpreters often use notes to help them remember what has been said. Unfortunately, note-taking can be a distractor to interpreters who have not practiced note-taking or do not take notes properly.

In this section, we will address the basics of how to practice taking notes and how to take notes properly.

HOW TO PRACTICE TAKING NOTES

The worst time to start practicing note-taking in a different way is during a live interpreting session. When interpreters are just starting out or changing their note-taking system, they will spend much of their attention on *how* to take notes instead of on the speaker's message.

> Interpreters (like all professionals) have a limited amount of attention and memory, so every bit of attention or memory spent on how to take notes inevitably distracts from understanding and remembering the speaker's message.

Therefore, some of the best ways to practice taking notes includes while listening to recordings and when practicing with other interpreters. Both of these methods allow the interpreter to pause, review, and repeat their practice without affecting medical outcomes.

HOW TO PROPERLY TAKE NOTES

Before anything else, the interpreter should ask for permission from the patient and provider to take notes during the session. The interpreter should explain that he/she will be taking notes to help remember everything that is said so that he/she can provide a complete and accurate interpretation. The interpreter should also reassure the patient that the notes will be destroyed after the end of the session (usually interpreters can give the notes to the provider afterward to be shredded).

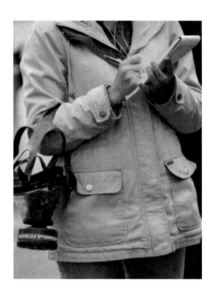

When taking notes, interpreters should only try to capture the main ideas of a message. Note-taking is not a replacement for an interpreter's memory. Instead, interpreters use notes to *help* them remember more information at a time and to make it easier to remember so they do not tire as quickly.

When you start taking notes, try to only write down three or four words per sentence. You should not worry at first about symbols and abbreviations. Just practice *what to write* instead of *how to write it*, so you will still be able to focus on the speaker's message.

Once you feel comfortable identifying the most important words or symbols to write down, you can start slowly developing your own personalized abbreviations and symbols for common terms and actions that you interpret.

WHAT TO AVOID WHEN BEGINNING NOTE-TAKING

Here are a few things to avoid when note-taking:

1. Before note-taking, do not forget to inform to all parties that you will be taking notes and that the notes will be discarded after the session.

2. Do not worry about making your notes look neat. Only you will decode your notes.

3. Do not worry about using too much paper. Use the space on the page to help you remember relationships, the order of events, and parts of speech.

4. If you do not know how to write down an idea, just focus on people, places, things, ideas, and actions. These are the central parts of almost any message.

5. Do not use shorthand unless you know it well.

6. Do not forget to discard your notes. They have no value after the assignment and misplacement could violate HIPAA.

19

EXPANDED NOTE-TAKING SKILLS

LEARNING GOAL

► After successful completion of the Expanded Note-Taking Skills chapter, participants will be able to be skilled at taking notes.

LEARNING OBJECTIVES:

Using the above goals, participants should also be able to do the following upon successful completion of this chapter:

► Understand and explain the needed skills for taking notes.
► Always write decontextualized information.
► Learn how to use Diagonal SVO Note-Taking.
► Learn how to use linking words.

IMPORTANT TERMS AND WORDS

► Decontextualized Information
► Diagonal SVO
► Linking Words

in confirming a telephone number, or proper spelling of a name, if you need to, in order to interpret it correctly, or if you foresee having to interpret that name more than once.

HOW TO USE DIAGONAL SVO NOTE-TAKING

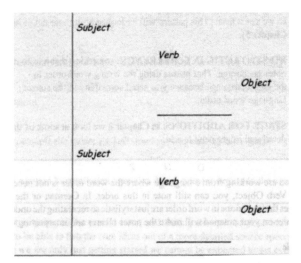

We have touched on how to take notes (writing down only the key ideas in each sentence) and how to avoid some common pitfalls. In this section, we will discuss decontextualized information, how to use diagonal SVO (subject-verb-object) note-taking, and linking words.

ALWAYS WRITE DECONTEXTUALIZED INFORMATION

CONTEXTUALIZATION means analyzing a word or event in terms of the words or concepts surrounding it. Contextualization aids memory and helps an interpreter understand a message.

Unfortunately, not all information can be placed in context. Some information such as names, addresses, and telephone numbers must be interpreted, but they are not connected to other parts of a story or message the same way that a description is.

Always write down decontextualized information in your notes. Decontextualized information is generally the hardest information to remember. Ask for confirmation, as

Interpreters with good note-taking habits tend to use a lot of space when taking notes. This is because space itself can have meaning. Interpreters generally start a sentence in the top left hand of a page and then note ideas in diagonal patterns. This arrangement makes it easier for interpreters to remember the parts of speech of the things they write.

In a common system of note-taking called **SVO note-taking**, interpreters place the subject of the sentence on the top left of the page, the verb in the middle of the page, and the object in the bottom right of the page. Using this system, interpreters can build on this system to describe subjects and objects by placing words in the right parts of the page or list actions or things without worrying about mixing them up with other parts of the sentence.

Because this system uses a lot of paper, many interpreters prefer to use notebooks that have a spiral on top such as a steno notebook because it is easier to quickly flip between pages with these notebooks.

HOW TO USE LINKING WORDS

Although there appear to be many linking words in English, many of them have similar meanings. Interpreters are much more concerned with meaning than with words themselves, so most interpreters combine similar terms when taking notes. One good example of this is the word "although." In English, some synonyms of "although"

include "albeit," "despite," "notwithstanding," "supposing," and "whereas." All of these ideas can be represented by the same symbol.

In fact, according to Andrew Gillies' well-regarded book *Note-Taking for Consecutive Interpreting*, all linking words can be reduced to the following list: "but," "although," "hence," "in order to," "if/then," "for example," and "in addition." By making a symbol for each of these terms and being aware of related linking words, interpreters can quickly link ideas in complex as well as simple sentences.

KEEP OUT THE OBVIOUS

Some words are not worth the trouble of writing down. For example, you can often skip verbs like "to be" and "there is/there are" entirely because the rest of the sentence will help you remember these verbs.

Likewise, if you are interpreting a story, don't worry too much about tenses. The context of the message will help you remember. Most of the events will be in an easily remembered past tense, and opinions will be contextualized in the past or present tense.

Additionally, sometimes you can reduce the number of notes you take when speakers mention related concepts. Often, speakers talk about opposites or synonyms when trying to explain something, but you generally only need to write one down in order to remember both since these ideas are already linked.

20

USING SYMBOLS WHEN NOTE-TAKING

LEARNING GOAL

► After successful completion of the Using Symbols when Note-Taking chapter, participants will be able to be skilled at using symbols when taking notes.

LEARNING OBJECTIVES:

Using the above goals, participants should also be able to do the following upon successful completion of this chapter:

► Understand and explain how to use symbols effectively when taking notes.
► Learn when to use symbols
► Learn how to design symbols.
► Understand how symbols are modifiable.
► Identify symbols as language neutral.
► Learn how to use letters or common medical abbreviations to aid their note-taking.

IMPORTANT TERMS AND WORDS

► Symbols
► Language Neutral
► Modifiable

► Biopsy
► Permanent recording

Symbols are ideas represented by a simple picture, shape, or marking. A symbol does not have to be a literal drawing of the thing it represents. Interpreters often use symbols when taking notes because, unlike abbreviations or words, symbols are modifiable and language neutral.

WHEN TO USE SYMBOLS

Consider using symbols for many different things: actions, job titles, places, ideas, relationships, and more. Once you start creating and using symbols in note-taking, the most difficult thing can be to pace yourself and adopt symbols slowly.

So, what things should you create symbols for first? Some of the best candidates for symbols are things that come up over and over again or terms that you have difficulty remembering. For example, if you often work in a dermatologist's office, you might consider making a symbol for "biopsy."

However, some words are not good candidates for symbols because they are generally not important enough to write down. Some examples include "a," "an," "the," and filler words such as "well," "umm," and "so".

HOW TO DESIGN SYMBOLS

No two interpreters use all the same symbols. The best way to make new symbols is by creating or choosing something that has meaning to you. When you create your own symbols, you put thought into the process that helps your brain to remember the symbol later. Even if you borrow another interpreter's symbol, you should consciously decide why you like that symbol so that your brain remembers the symbol later when you need it.

One word of caution: symbols are a memory tool, not a permanent recording. Do not waste time making your symbols elaborate, neat, or fully explanatory. You only need symbols to assist your short-term memory, not to be read by archaeologists in the far future.

Likewise, do not forget to practice drawing your symbols so that your hand will be familiar with the motion and be able to complete the symbol faster. Many beginning interpreters make the mistake of taking longer to draw symbols than it would take them to write out the word. Avoid falling into this trap by drawing the symbol several times and actively thinking about how to further simplify it when you are interpreting.

HOW SYMBOLS ARE MODIFIABLE

One other advantage of symbols is that they are modifiable. Consider that in English a single concept can have many different variations according to number, tense, and parts of speech. For example, the word "build" can also be "building(s) (noun and participle)," built," "built up," and "over built."

Instead of making a separate symbol for each of these words, you can simply add to or modify (change) your symbol to reflect the specific meaning. In this case, you might use the symbol of a hammer (which you can simplify with a sideways triangle and line beneath) for "build" and add an exclamation point for "building," an arrow for "built up," or a line over the hammer for "over built."

SYMBOLS ARE LANGUAGE NEUTRAL

Using a common medical interpreting example, the word "surgery" can be represented by an angle symbol (representing a knife) and a square (representing a body).

This symbol is *language neutral* because it is not specific to the English representation of this concept. The knife and body would be an equally recognizable symbol in Spanish, for example.

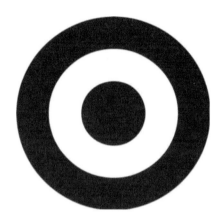

LETTERS AND COMMON MEDICAL ABBREVIATIONS

In addition to symbols, interpreters can use letters or common medical abbreviations to aid their note-taking. Here are some examples of commonly used short-hands in medical interpreting:

Treatment	Rx	Without	S
History	Hx	With	C
Diagnosis	Ox	If needed	sos
Every	q	Before meals	AC
Everyday	qd	After meals	PC
Every other day	qod	Twice a day	B I D
Every hour	qh	Trice a day	T I D
Every morning	QAM	Four times a day	Q I d
Every 4 hours	Q 4 H	Once a day	O D
As needed	PRN	Twice a week	TW
At bed time	H S	Before Breakfast	BBF
By mouth; orally	PO	Before dinner	BD
milligram	MG	Ounce	OZ
kilogram	KG	Cups	C
Gram	G	Pounds	lb
Teaspoon	tsp	Tablespoon	tbs
degrees Fahrenheit	F	milliliter	ML
degrees centigrade/Celsius	C	Liter	L
Number	# OR no.	Page	pg
Year	YR	At	@
Month	mth	Following	ff
Per	/	Maximum	max

Less than	<	Minimum	min
More than	>	Most importantly	*
Question	Q	Answer	A
Problem	prob	Equals	=
Before	b/4	Word	wd
Percent	%	Because	b/c
Versus /against	vs	With	w/
Department	Dept	Without	w/o
Within	w/i	Reference	ref

21

BASIC SKILLS IN SIGHT TRANSLATION

LEARNING GOAL

► After successful completion of the Basic Skills in Sight Translation chapter, participants will be able to learn how sight translate documents during their medical interpreting encounter.

LEARNING OBJECTIVES:

Using the above goals, participants should also be able to do the following upon successful completion of this chapter:

► Understand and explain the needed basic skills in sight translation.
► Compare sight translation and consecutive mode.
► Learn the needed 5 steps to sight translation.
► Know the importance of taking your time when sight translating.
► Learn how and what to take notes for when sight translating.

IMPORTANT TERMS AND WORDS

► Long pauses
► Potential pitfalls
► Language patterns
► Continuous pace

► Segments
► Macro-unit
► Diagonal SVO

Sight translation is the third mode of interpreting after consecutive and simultaneous interpreting.

Sight translation occurs when an interpreter verbally reads a text in a language different than the one the message is written in. In sight translation, no written translation is provided (this is the work of translators, not interpreters).

Interpreters should perform sight translation only for short documents. In general, you should not sight translate a document you do not understand well or that is more than two pages long.

COMPARING SIGHT TRANSLATION AND CONSECUTIVE MODE

Whereas consecutive mode commonly uses short messages with pauses, allows for note-taking while listening, and does not contain long pauses, sight translation is the opposite.

With sight translation, interpreters speak for a long period at a time with pauses in between units of interpreting.

Sight translation is also quite different from written translation. Whereas written translation allows for significant delays to find the exact right term or phrase, sight translation must be prepared quickly.

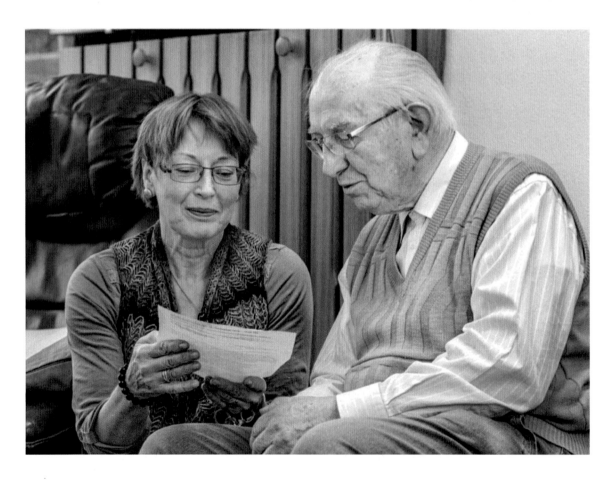

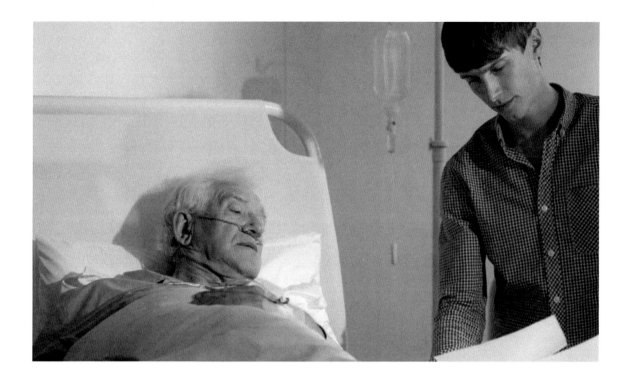

5 STEPS TO SIGHT TRANSLATION

Almost every interpreter will have to refuse a sight translation at some point either because the document to be sight translated is too long or too complex. If it is too long, the interpreter must request that it be translated for the patient. However, when you are able to sight translate, follow these five steps:

1. Silently read the document all the way through;

2. Identify unfamiliar concepts and potential pitfalls;

3. Analyze the register and language patterns;

4. Ask for clarification if needed; and

5. Read at a steady, moderate, continuous pace.

THE IMPORTANCE OF TAKING YOUR TIME

It can feel awkward to take several minutes to silently read a document in the middle of an interpreting session, but you should take the time you need to prepare so that you will not have to pause again to read ahead in the middle of the document. Providers and LEP persons may show signs of impatience if you take longer than they expect, but you should explain if necessary that you are taking time to preview the document so that you will be able to sight translate the whole document at once. Sometimes asking to leave the room to study the document takes away the pressure of having two people over one's shoulder waiting for you to read the text. Ask for a pencil or pen to mark the document with your notes if that helps so that when you are sight translating you can do it with greater ease.

In summary, it is very important to read the entire document first. If you do not read the document before beginning sight translation, you will not be familiar with its contents, and will need to pause or correct yourself more. Pauses and corrections are confusing to the listener during sight translation because they cannot see the structure of the document, so it sounds like parts of information are coming in bits and pieces. Unlike in spoken language, the organization of written titles, headings, and paragraphs signals to readers how each sentence relates to each other. Therefore, if you pause while reading the document, the listener is more likely not to understand. Generally, it is better to do a longer pause before each sentence, read it, and then interpret it into segments. If you just interpret segments, the entire text reads like a series of continuous segments. The longer pause aids the listener to understand that a sentence, or macro-unit of message, is finished and another one will start soon. It is also good to explain or interpret what you see as you sight translate. For example, an interpreter may state, "This is a new section entitled: How to Prepare for Your Surgery".

NOTE-TAKING FOR SIGHT TRANSLATION

When taking notes for sight-translation, do not use regular diagonal SVO (subject-verb-object) notes. Instead, write down words or phrases that you need to pay special attention to and, if necessary, write the target language term(s) or expression(s) you will use.

> If appropriate, ask the provider whether you can mark the document. Marking the document, especially by circling, or underlining words and phrases, will greatly speed up your ability to create a mini-glossary on the spot.

If you are unsure about the meaning of a sentence or term, ask the provider. Write down any answers the provider gives about a term to help you remember when sight translating.

NOTES

22

SPECIAL PROBLEMS WITH SIGHT TRANSLATION

LEARNING GOAL

► After successful completion of the Special Problems with Sight Translation chapter, participants will be able to learn how to manage sight translation and deal with all the special problems with sight translation.

LEARNING OBJECTIVES:

Using the above goals, participants should also be able to do the following upon successful completion of this chapter:

► Understand the special problems related to sight translation.

► Know how to address sight translation in pre-sessions or pre-conferences.

► Realize when to refuse to sight translate.

► Explain the five steps to refuse sight translations.

► Understand the importance of transparency when sight translating.

IMPORTANT TERMS AND WORDS

► Mini-glossary

► Effective. Advocating

► Justifiable reason

► Intake form

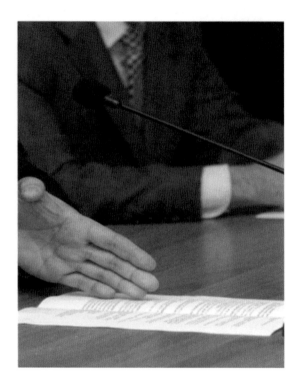

I n an ideal world, providers would always have written translations ready of any documents they needed to give to patients. However, that is often not the case.

In this section, we will cover some concerns that come up with sight translation that are unlikely to occur with other modes of interpreting.

ADDRESSING SIGHT TRANSLATION IN PRE-SESSIONS OR PRE-CONFERENCES

One great way to anticipate sight translations is to ask about them in a pre-conference. If you have an opportunity to have a pre-conference with the provider, you should also try to educate him or her about alternatives to sight translation such as verbal explanations or written translations

so as to reduce the amount of sight translations you may need to do in the future.

In a pre-session or pre-conference, you may also be able to take additional time to "pre-read" documents you will have to sight translate. If you have this opportunity, use your time to create a mini-glossary and think about the organization and language the document uses.

As a reminder, *always refuse sight translation requests that are too long or too complex.* Cite the reasons for doing so in a polite and professional manner. Usually providing explanations related to the patient's need to understand the document fully are very effective. Advocating for the document to be translated for the patient's safety and ability to reread if necessary is also a justifiable reason.

WHEN NOT TO SIGHT TRANSLATE

Do not sight translate documents that are too long, too complex, full of unfamiliar terminology, or otherwise beyond the ability of the interpreter to competently sight translate.

Also, be careful with documents that are used to write down a client's information such as an intake form. These documents should be read aloud to the patients and the patient will fill out this intake form.

THE FIVE STEPS TO REFUSE SIGHT TRANSLATIONS

One of the most important problem-solving skills in sight translation is to know how to refuse inappropriate requests, for example, when a document is more than two pages in length, has complex language, or is a legal document such as a consent to surgery.

When refusing a sight translation, follow these five easy steps:

First, do not say "no". However, you can say" I would love to do that" or "Thank you very much for trusting me". Remember that most providers do not like to hear the word "NO". They might think that you are challenging them, especially if they have asked other interpreters to do that and the interpreters accepted and for some reason did not refuse the task.

Second, say "but ". The word "but" negates or cancels what you already said earlier. So, you say that you cannot do that. Remember, although declining a request and saying "no" takes courage, it is an important professional skill.

Third, explain yourself and say why you cannot do what you are asked to do. You should mention some convincing reasons for your refusal based on your experience in this profession. Most of the time, the explanation will have to do with the document's length or content. *For example, "This document contains a lot of complicated terms that are beyond my linguistic abilities".* Or, "This document is full of complex medical terminology that requires terminological research and preparation, and the patient is unlikely to understand the sight translation, since I cannot pause when sight translating" or "unfortunately, this document is simply too long for a professional interpreter to sight translate; it needs to be translated for the patient."

Even simple reasons like "this document is too complex" work fine.

Fourth, reassure the provider that you would like to work as one team because you are part of the medical team. You can politely let the provider know that you are willing to do whatever you can to help them. For example, "I am ready to do whatever it takes to help you, but.."

Fifth, offer alternatives or solutions so that the provider knows what he or she can do instead of pushing you to sight translate. Examples of some alternatives include:

► Asking the provider to mark a portion of the document that he or she wants sight translated and showing the patient the portion that is being sight translated;

► Asking the provider to explain the document or have a nurse explain it;

► Suggesting that the provider obtain a written translation, where appropriate; or

► Requesting that the provider simplify the document so that it can be accurately sight-translated.

(taken in part from the Language of Justice: Interpreting for Legal Services course by Cross Cultural Communications)

Doctors are highly educated professionals, and they often do not realize when documents are written in a high register. Nevertheless, high-register language will often confuse patients because written language often uses longer sentences than spoken communication.

SIGHT TRANSLATE THE ENTIRE DOCUMENT

When sight translating, *do not lower the register*. Authors often choose their wording for a reason.

Remember to translate the ENTIRE document, including document titles, headings, address lines, and letterhead, and even signatures. You may feel silly sight translating these portions, but if you omit anything without telling both parties, you are not being transparent nor are you interpreting completely.

As mentioned previously, interpreters can ask providers in a pre-session to mark portions of a document to read and then explain to the patient that only part of the document is being sight translated.

TRANSPARENCY WHEN SIGHT TRANSLATING

If you skip any part of a document (e.g. at a provider's request), you must let both parties know. If one party interrupts to make a comment or ask a question, you will need to pause to interpret and let the provider know where you stopped sight translating.

Both parties must understand when you are sight translating the document and when you are interpreting a question or comment.

NOTES

23

CULTURE

LEARNING GOAL

► After successful completion of the Culture chapter, participants will be able to learn a lot about culture and how to manage culture challenges during the medical interpreting encounter.

LEARNING OBJECTIVES:

Using the above goals, participants should also be able to do the following upon successful completion of this chapter:

► Understand and explain cross-cultural competence and interpreting.
► Learn how to overcome cultural blind spots.
► Understand and illustrate the culture of biomedicine.

IMPORTANT TERMS AND WORDS

► Culture of Biomedicine
► Cultural Blind Spots
► Cross-Cultural Competence
► Cultural sensitivity
► Context

► Linguistic groups
► Ethnicity
► Caesarian Section (C-section)
► Surgical procedure
► Protocols

REVIEW OF CULTURE

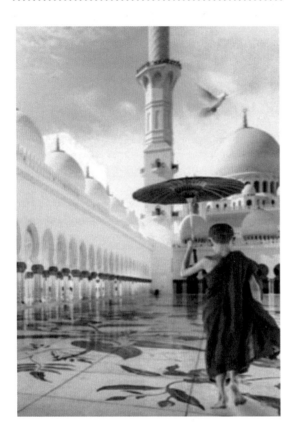

CULTURE is the context in which we view our relationships with family, partners, society, the world, and ourselves. This includes beliefs, traditions, and behaviors which an individual may not even be aware of. Although different groups share culture (linguistic groups, countries, clubs, gender groups, and professional groups), culture is ultimately individual to each person. In other words, even though many people in a group may share similar cultures, no two persons' culture is exactly the same, as so many factors will influence one's culture (ethnicity, family, relationships, education, environment, etc.).

CROSS-CULTURAL COMPETENCE AND INTERPRETING

As a medical interpreter or aspiring medical interpreter, you are sure to encounter persons and providers from many cultures who do not share their language or culture. Usually the interpreter has some knowledge of cultural nuances by the simple virtue of knowing the language. However, sometimes, you may be unfamiliar with one or more of these cultures, as culture is an individual phenomenon.

> Whenever interpreters encounter persons or providers from cultures with which they are unfamiliar, interpreters should be aware of the cultural assumptions they make by using a skill called cross-cultural competence.

CROSS-CULTURAL COMPETENCE OR CULTURAL SENSITIVITY refers to the knowledge, skills, and attitudes an interpreter adopts that help him or her to be sensitive, respectful, mindful, and adapt effectively with individuals of different cultures.

In general, interpreters who are cross-culturally competent recognize and value diversity among people. They try to understand other people's point of view, and they do not assume that there is only one right way to view themselves and others, nor that there is one right way to live.

This requires that interpreters be open to different ideas and beliefs and be able to agree to disagree in many aspects of life.

Unfortunately, even interpreters with high levels of cross-cultural competence have some **cultural blind spots**, which are unconscious biases towards a culture—or part of a culture—which an interpreter dislikes or of which he or she is unaware.

These are aspects of another culture of which an interpreter is unaware or that he or she ignores. Try to regularly be aware of cultural blind spots and identify new ones as you gain experience in the interpreting field.

HOW TO OVERCOME CULTURAL BLIND SPOTS

The first rule for overcoming cultural blind spots is to be attentive to other people's reactions when interpreting. Interpreters should look at a person's nonverbal messages in their posture, facial expressions, tone of voice, and body language. Nonverbal messages are as important as verbal messages. It is also important to be attentive to the verbal messages, hesitations, emphasis, and other paralinguistic (beyond language) features, to judge how that person might feel or how he or she is reacting to what is happening.

Next, be adaptive. While interpreters will not intervene in the interpreted conversation unless necessary, an interpreter can use his or her positioning, tone of voice, and hand signals to make the parties feel more comfortable.

When the need to intervene is identified, interpreters must rely on their cross-cultural competence to identify and resolve cultural barriers.

THE CULTURE OF BIOMEDICINE

The Western medicine system, or biomedicine, is a system in which medical doctors and other healthcare professionals (such as nurses, pharmacists, and therapists) treat symptoms and diseases using drugs, radiation, or surgery. Medical doctors in different parts of the world have many things in common. For example, doctors in Jordan, India, and the United States all may use an X-ray machine to find out if a child with a hurt leg has broken a bone. However, doctors in other parts of the world can also be very different from the US and other countries. For example, in Brazil over half of babies are born by Caesarian Section (C-section), a surgical procedure to remove a baby from the uterus. In the United States, doctors perform this procedure much less often.

While some of the differences in medical practice between countries have to do with the education and resources available to doctors in each country, much of the difference can be explained by the medical cultures of each country. Below we look into some habits, beliefs, protocols, and rules that doctors and other medical staff follow in the United States.

BIOMEDICAL CULTURE

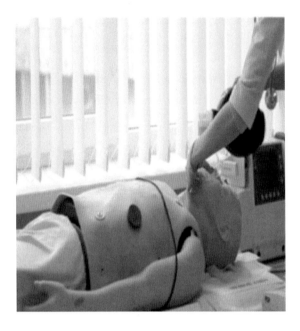

A **biomedical culture** involves the expectations, habits, beliefs, protocols, and rules people have about healthcare and the relationships between doctors, medical staff, and patients. Biomedical culture is one of the biggest reasons why doctors in different areas often diagnose and treat patients differently.

In the United States, most doctors focus on diseases, symptoms, disabilities or the rehabilitation of patients. This is known as the **biomedical model of medicine**. It is also called allopathic medicine, biomedicine, conventional medicine, mainstream medicine, and orthodox medicine.

In the United States, doctors who use this model will diagnose the problem and then negotiate with the patient the best treatment to pursue. Each person in the interpreted communicative event has their sphere of expertise. The doctor is the expert and in charge of inquiring, locating and understanding the problem and identifying the possible solutions, if any. The patient is the ultimate expert in their own body and is in charge of explaining his or her symptoms to the best of their ability in order to receive treatment. The patient also has the responsibility to participate in their healing by complying with the agreed treatment plan. The interpreter is the ultimate expert in interpreting language/culture and in the process of intercultural communication. The interpreter is responsible for mediating the communication between patient and provider in an accurate, transparent and ethical manner.

One major difference between the biomedical model of medicine and other models (such as Alternative Medicine, to be discussed later) is that doctors rarely consider the effects of psychological, environmental, and social influences on the patient. Instead, based on the doctor's training and the practicalities of practicing medicine in a capitalistic society, the focus of the doctor is to treat the disease in the most efficient manner. The provider-patient interaction and relationship is professionally oriented (objective and purpose-oriented, versus personal). The purpose for the patient is to tell the doctor what the complaint is, and for the doctor the purpose is to find the problem and treat it. However, doctors cannot do everything in a treatment. If a doctor prescribes medication, it will only work if the patient takes the medication exactly as prescribed. Therefore, it is recognized in the United States that the patient has an important role in their own healing.

24

BODY LANGUAGE AND CULTURE

LEARNING GOAL

► After successful completion of the Body Language and Culture chapter, participants will be able to learn how to manage interpreting the body language of any party when facilitating understanding in the communication between the patient and the provider.

LEARNING OBJECTIVES:

Using the above goals, participants should also be able to do the following upon successful completion of this chapter:

► Understand and explain how to manage interpreting body language that is related to the culture of the speaker.
► Learn how to deal with the gender and biological sex issues when interpreting.
► Learn the best way to address all parties during the medical encounter.

IMPORTANT TERMS AND WORDS

► Gender and biological sex
► Body language
► Formal address
► Facial expression,
► Hand gesture
► Transgender

► Risking offense
► Female characteristics
► Modesty,
► Chaperones
► Cohabitation
► Patient's autonomy

Even in cases where the meaning of a facial expression, hand gesture or body movement may seem clear, the interpreter should not assume they know the meaning, and instead, let the parties try to navigate the communication on their own. This way, the provider and patient can establish better trust by learning to communicate and deal with their issues directly with each other.

If necessary, interpreters can ask one party to confirm the meaning of a certain body language. The interpreter will never ask a patient to explain why they look worried or why they seem nervous. That would be an odd request. It is easier and more practical and realistic to intervene and tell the provider the interpreter needs to ask the patient or simply ask the patient if they are nervous as the interpreter is reading body language that seems to say so.

or another gender. For a majority of people, their gender is the same as their biological sex. However, for some individuals, gender and biological sex are different.

Persons with a gender different than their biological sex are often referred to as **transgender**. When interpreting, be sure to not disrespect a transgender person by using the wrong linguistic gender to refer to him or her. Instead, always use a person's preferred gender if that person states their gender.

Sometimes, interpreters may not be certain which gender to use when referring to a patient or medical provider. In such a case, interpreters should ask "what gender pronoun should I use to address you" instead of risking offense by using the wrong gender for a party.

Remember: when in doubt, ask politely and always use a person's preferred gender.

GENDER

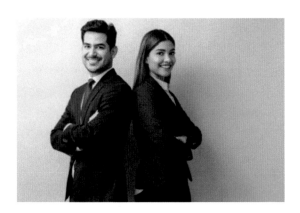

GENDER, unlike biological sex, is the identity a person holds regarding being male, female,

BIOLOGICAL SEX

In contrast from gender, a person's **biological sex** refers to male or female characteristics that a person's body has.

Cultures vary widely in their attitudes towards biological sex, including attitudes about jobs, public and private space, modesty, chaperones, dating, friendships, conversation, cohabitation, and professional relationships between people of another sex.

Not all cultures have just male and female sexes, and not all people are easily identified as only male or female. In medicine, a person with internal genitalia that do not match that person's external genitalia is an **intersex** person. When interpreting for intersex persons, be aware of the need to respect that person's preferred pronouns as explained in the "Gender" subsection above.

FORMAL ADDRESS

FORMAL ADDRESS is the use of more respectful, professional, less intimate/personal way of referring to a person you are talking to.

Interpreters should almost always use a professional, formal address in interpreting unless there is a strong reason not to do so. Some common exceptions include speaking to children or persons with disabilities who may be confused by the use of a formal address.

Some interpreters may feel that using a formal address is inappropriate in the cultural context in which they work. However, please note that a more formal address avoids the appearance of a patient being or feeling like an interpreter's personal friend. Using a formal form of address with patients is a good way of ensuring that patients understand the professional relationship or distance that needs to be there between patient and interpreter for objectivity and neutrality. However, there are cases where a formal form of address may make the patient uncomfortable. In these cases, interpreters should speak with colleagues who share the same or similar language pairs or cultural issues to determine the best solution. You should generally not use a term that would make a patient feel like he or she is not empowered to make his or her own medical decisions. Remember the patient's autonomy which means that the patient is the only one who decides for themselves and the interpreters should not decide for them or suggest any solutions for them.

When in doubt, use formal, respectful language for all parties.

The interpreters should not mimic the providers who might address patients informally, for example by addressing the LEP by their first name. Instead, interpreters should use a more formal form to uphold respect and cultural sensitivity.

25

SWEAR-WORDS, OBSCENITIES, BODY PARTS, AND MODESTY

LEARNING GOAL

► After successful completion of the Swear-Words, Obscenities, Body Parts, and Modesty chapter, participants will be able to learn a lot about the providers and LEP patients' culture of swear-words, obscenities, body parts and modesty. And how they can manage interpreting all of them.

LEARNING OBJECTIVES:

Using the above goals, participants should also be able to do the following upon successful completion of this chapter:

► Learn how to interpret vulgarities.
► Learn how to effectively manage overcoming the embarrassment of terminology references to sex acts or bodily functions that can be cultural taboos.
► Learn how to interpret humor during the medical encounter.
► Illustrate how to play their role as a cultural broker effectively.

IMPORTANT TERMS AND WORDS

- ► Swear-Words,
- ► Obscenities
- ► Vulgarities
- ► A judgmental statement
- ► Linguistic equivalent
- ► Interpretation rendition
- ► References to sex acts
- ► Cultural taboo
- ► Communicative autonomy
- ► An interpreting distortion
- ► Humor

- ► Linguistic differences
- ► Cultural concept
- ► Circular vs. linear
- ► Reserved vs. expressive
- ► Consensus-driven,
- ► Intuitive
- ► Orientation
- ► Flexible vs. rigid
- ► Childrearing or childbearing
- ► Intercultural humility
- ► Diversity of opinions

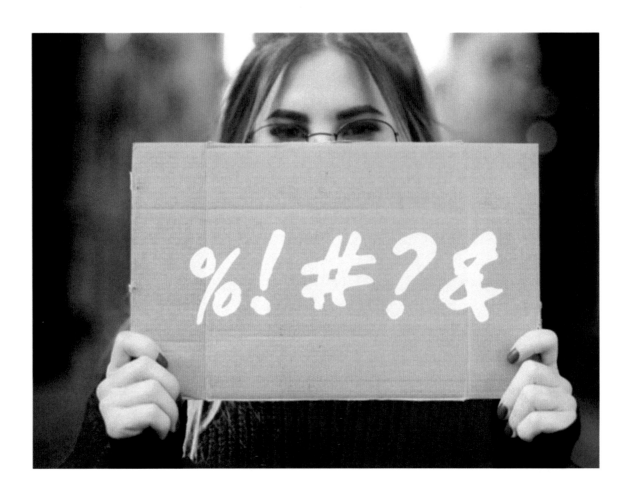

SWEAR-WORDS

Interpreters often struggle with expressing vulgarities they may feel are embarrassing or morally wrong. However, an interpreter's job is to communicate the speaker's message as completely and accurately as possible. Interpreters have a professional (and ethical) responsibility to interpret even things they may personally think are wrong. Interpreters need to remember that these are not their messages. Personal objections have no place in a professional setting. When the interpreter is acting as a professional, he has to forget about his personal or cultural opinions or beliefs and act as a neutral and impartial agent of communication. Remember the tip to learn to agree to disagree? It is not up to the interpreter to censor either party.

Aside from personal objections, swear-words can be difficult because they may not have direct translations. If you do not know the meaning of a swear-word, *do not guess* and do not simply explain that the patient "said something inappropriate", which would be a judgmental statement. Instead, use problem-solving to clarify the meaning just as you would with any other term.

In cases where there simply is not a linguistic equivalent for the swear-word, the best action to take is to ask the speaker what the word means and then interpret the speaker's explanation, even if the interpreter already knows the meaning. This way, the interpreter avoids inserting his or her opinion into the interpretation rendition.

OBSCENITIES, BODY PARTS, AND MODESTY

For many interpreters, references to sex acts or bodily functions can also be cultural taboo. However, interpreters need to be professional at all times and overcome embarrassment with terminology. Interpreters who inject their personal cultural beliefs into a session are not culturally competent to interpret. Interpreting is a profession that requires one to interpret everything that is said, without objection. *Remember that you are not speaking with your own voice. If you absolutely cannot interpret the words that are used, you must withdraw from the assignment. However, be advised that you may not be called often to interpret.*

Interpreting even obscene words is important because patients deserve to have communicative autonomy, or independence, which means that the speaker's voice is not changed (including tone, word-choice, style, and register) in the target language. This would encompass an interpreting distortion.

INTERPRETING HUMOR

Humor is also very closely tied to culture. Some jokes can be replaced with an equivalent, which requires quick thinking on the part of the interpreter, but simply do not have a linguistic equivalent.

If the joke will make sense in the target language, the interpreter should simply interpret it as normal. However, when the joke will be confusing or strange to the other party, the interpreter will have to problem-solve.

For example, there are times when an interpreter must simply report that the speaker said something that is amusing but that cannot be interpreted because of linguistic differences.

When interpreting humor, keep in mind the speaker's style, tone, and use of offensive language, if any.

There are several challenges to cultural mediation or being a cultural broker:

First, when interpreters perform intercultural mediation, there is a possibility that the party will not understand the issue, as a cultural concept may be known or understood by one party but be difficult to understand for another. This means that the interpreter needs to know what types of cultural issues typically arise. The most common intercultural differences involve:

1. Communication style (circular vs. linear)

2. Decision-making (individual, linear vs. consensus-driven, intuitive)

3. Expression (reserved vs. expressive)

4. Orientation (group vs. individual)

5. Level of commitment to relationships (high vs. low)

6. Sense of time (flexible vs. rigid)

7. Relationships (many, looser, short-term vs. fewer, tighter, long-term)

8. Childrearing or childbearing beliefs

9. Role of the elderly in society

Sometimes there are two conflicting cultural assumptions or views of the same issue. The IMIA Standard of Practice (IMIA: A-12), states that the interpreter needs to be able to "manage conflict between the provider and the patient". However, this does not mean the interpreter needs to resolve the conflict. The IMIA provides the following steps to address a conflict:

A. Remain calm in stressful situations or when there is a conflict.

B. Acknowledge when there is conflict or tension between provider and patient.

C. Assist the provider and patient in making conflicts or tensions explicit (known), so that they can work them out between themselves.

D. Let the parties speak for themselves and do not take sides in the conflict.

Cultural mediation occurs more often when there is a greater cultural gap between a patient and a provider, or if the patient comes from a cultural background that the provider may not understand well or have regular contact with.

A WORD ABOUT CULTURAL INTERVENTION

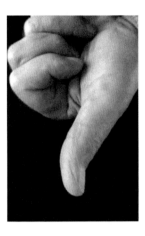

Intervention to remove a cultural barrier is often much more complicated than intervention to remove a linguistic barrier, so interpreters should be extra cautious. A person's culture is often highly individualized, and interpreters should use appropriate messaging when they address issues related to the patient's or provider's culture. The interpreters should strive not to offend or stereotype anyone or create a new stereotype.

An example of good cultural mediation (cultural broker role) might be to address the fact that people in some cultures put their hands to their hearts or simply bow instead of shaking hands. If a provider is confused, the interpreter could quickly intervene and transparently let the parties know what is happening (e.g. "[patient] is putting his/her hand to his/her heart to return your handshake"). The interpreter should always remember to intervene and play this role, cultural mediator (Cultural Broker) in both languages.

Of course, interpreters first need to be very familiar with a specific group culture before performing cultural mediation (problem solving). Interpreters who do not know enough about the multiple cultures of their interpreting languages should constantly work to expand their knowledge and have cultural humility and cultural curiosity to be able to remove these cultural barriers whenever they appear. There needs to be cultural humility, since even if one is very familiar with a specific group culture, one cannot assume to know the cultural background of that specific patient or provider, since each individual has a unique cultural makeup that is only partially influenced by their country or regional culture. Other factors influence one's cultural makeup, such as educational background, being of a rural or urban background, age, personal experiences, and several other factors.

Additionally, it is important to note that the intercultural mediation role is not always about explaining a cultural issue about the patient's culture to the provider or addressing a cultural issue that may affect understanding. Intercultural mediation is also about explaining something about biomedical culture or American culture to the patient. For example, often patients are surprised to be asked if they consume alcohol, or if they do drugs. When the interpreter notices a non-verbal message of discomfort with these questions, the interpreter may decide to alert the patient that in the US all providers have to ask these questions to all patients by law. This helps the patient not feel that he or she is being singled out, by giving context to the message. Or, interpreters may need to explain to the family about HIPAA and why the provider cannot speak to them until he or she obtains expressed permission from the patient. Otherwise, the family may lose trust in the provider. Interpreters should be mindful to balance their intercultural mediation in both directions for the benefit of the therapeutic rapport and to increase impartiality. If an interpreter is only working one way, it leaves the other party uninformed as to what they also need to know to be more culturally knowledgeable. Keep in mind, mediation is an impartial activity and is different from being someone's educator. It has to go both ways in order for the interpreter to be valued as a cultural agent in the system, and not just as a patient's cultural representative.

. . . .

Last, self-knowledge is very key in intercultural humility and awareness. One needs to understand their own cultural values well, how they relate or compare with other opposing cultural values, and learn to respect and appreciate diversity of opinions and traditions.

. . . .

NOTES

26

US HEALTHCARE SYSTEM

LEARNING GOAL

► After successful completion of the US Healthcare System chapter, participants will be able to have a full understanding of the US Healthcare system and the laws related to healthcare system and LEP patients.

LEARNING OBJECTIVES:

Using the above goals, participants should also be able to do the following upon successful completion of this chapter:

► Understand and explain the US healthcare system and its laws.

► Learn the Equal Access to Care laws.

► Learn the Roles of Doctors, Nurses, and Other Staff.

► Fully understand and explain the Patient Privacy HIPAA.

► Know important interpreting medical terminology to help participants during medical interpreting encounters.

IMPORTANT TERMS AND WORDS

- ► Equal Access to Care
- ► Title VI of the 1964 Civil Rights Act
- ► Ground of race, color, or national origin
- ► Denied the benefits
- ► Discrimination
- ► Federal financial assistance
- ► ADA (Americans with Disabilities Act),
- ► Culturally and Linguistically Appropriate Services (CLAS).

- ► Pharmacists
- ► Nurse Practitioners
- ► Direct supervision
- ► Patient Privacy HIPAA
- ► Health Insurance Portability and Accountability Act
- ► Consent
- ► Medicaid
- ► PT physical therapist

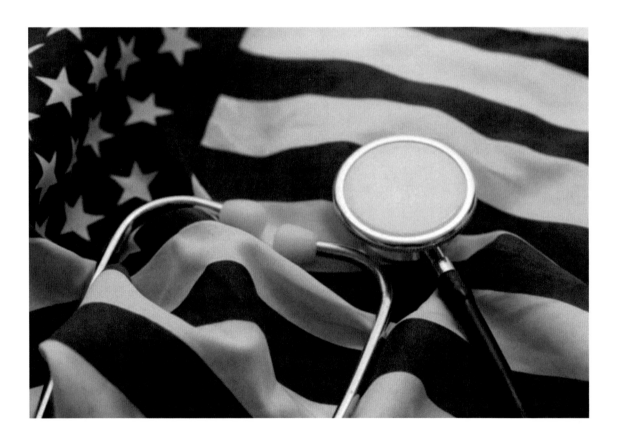

Although medical doctors practice all over the world have a lot of similarity but there are a lot of differences in medical practice between countries that have to do with the education and resources available to doctors in each country, much of the difference can be explained by the medical cultures of each country. Below we look into some habits, beliefs, and rules that doctors and other medical staff follow in the United States.

EQUAL ACCESS TO CARE

Most healthcare providers have an obligation in the United States to provide interpreters for LEP persons because of several laws that mandate equal access to health services. The best-known of these laws is known as Title VI of the Civil Rights Act of 1964. The Title VI of the Civil Rights Act of 1964 specifically says, "no person in the United States shall, on the ground of race, color, or national origin, be excluded from participation in, be denied the benefits of, or be subjected to discrimination under any program or activity receiving Federal financial assistance."

Virtually all healthcare facilities in the United States receive federal financial assistance, so in your professional work it is safe to assume that Title VI applies unless a provider or agency shows you otherwise. Most important to interpreters regarding Title VI of the 1964 Civil Rights Act is that it prohibits discrimination in healthcare settings on the basis of national origin, which includes a patient's language.

Sign language interpreters should also be aware of the ADA (Americans with Disabilities Act), which requires healthcare providers (among many others) to provide sign-language interpreters to deaf and hard of hearing patients.

The ADA (Americans with Disabilities Act) and Civil Rights Act are far from the only laws that influence interpreting in healthcare, but they are the best starting point for interpreters to be familiar with. Interpreters seeking to expand their knowledge of the legal framework surrounding interpreting in healthcare settings may also consult the Department of Health and Human Services Standards for Culturally and Linguistically Appropriate Services (CLAS).

THE ROLES OF DOCTORS, NURSES, AND OTHER STAFF

In the United States, healthcare providers are usually certified and licensed to practice. In most states, no one is allowed to practice medicine without a license.

MEDICAL DOCTORS (also called physicians, or MDs) are the only professionals who can treat patients. They can refer patients to specialists and write prescriptions.

SPECIALIZED PHYSICIANS are physicians that only practice medicine in a particular specialty (pediatrician, gastroenterologist, urologist, etc.)

SURGEONS are the only medical professionals that can authorize and perform surgery.

PHARMACISTS are professionally qualified to prepare and dispense medicinal drugs.

NURSES are licensed healthcare professionals who care for the sick or infirm under the supervision of a doctor or a nurse manager.

NURSE PRACTITIONERS are nurses who have additional practitioner education (master's degree or doctoral degrees such as DNP or PhD), and can treat certain medical conditions and prescribe medications without the direct supervision of a doctor.

(NOTE: They are not the same as a specialized nurse nor are they the same as physician assistants.)

Sometimes, patients get confused about what type of professional they have spoken with and what that person's role was. When interpreting, make sure that the patient knows who you are and what your role is. According to The Joint Commission (an organization that accredits hospitals based on patient safety measures), every patient must know at all times who is treating/working with them and what their role is.

PATIENT PRIVACY HIPAA

In many countries, but especially in the US, where privacy is a strong cultural value, patient information is kept private from everyone except for the **treating team** (the doctors, staff, and interpreters) and the patient. The main law that controls patient confidentiality (privacy) is called **HIPAA**, which stands for the Health Insurance Portability and Accountability Act. The Health and Human Services Department has very useful information and videos about HIPAA for all healthcare workers (see: https://www.hhs.gov/hipaa/index.html).

Patients have always had the right to access their own medical information, but HIPAA protects that information from others, due to concerns it will be used against the patient. For example, healthcare providers may not give any health information about a patient to family members unless the patient gives expressed **consent** (gives expressed permission). Many family members, therefore, feel confused when a family member's doctor or interpreter will not talk to them about their patient. In these cases, it is up to the interpreter to explain to them that in the United States there are privacy laws that do not allow the doctor to speak to them unless the patient requests so. It is possible that the doctor will not realize that the patient may have a different experience or laws in their home country.

PRIVATE HEALTHCARE

In the US, there is a public healthcare system that is designated for individuals from low-income backgrounds (Medicaid) and for elderly people over the age of 65 (Medicare). Private healthcare is healthcare that is paid by the patient, by the healthcare insurance company, or by both. In private healthcare, doctors are not supposed to turn patients away from emergency services based on inability to pay. Some patients may be worried about their ability to pay for healthcare in case of emergency, or they may be confused about what their health insurance will pay for.

On the other hand, doctors will turn away patients if they cannot pay their portion of fees for routine care. This applies to both children and adults. Patients with insurance may be required to pay the entire fee until they meet a *deductible*, or they may be responsible for a *co-pay (patient's portion of the payment for the service)*, both of which may be strange concepts to a patient, particularly if he or she is not from the United States. The interpreter should be able to clarify that to the patient and educate them about the healthcare insurance laws and regulations through the help of the providers.

In summary, when interpreting in healthcare, always be aware of the possibility of misguided patient expectations regarding payment, privacy, or the roles of different healthcare workers.

AN IMPORTANT OBSERVATION ABOUT INTERPRETING MEDICAL TERMINOLOGY:

Doctors use many acronyms, or abbreviations. PT is physical therapist, but when a physical therapist states to a patient that he or she is a PT, it is important for the interpreter to interpret the meaning, and not the words. Therefore, the interpreter will interpret PT as 'physical therapist' and not the letters, 'PT', which does not mean physical therapist in most languages. Please keep this in mind when you are interpreting. Our role plays will include these abbreviations. Remember to interpret their meaning and not simply repeat letters such as, 'PT'; that will not mean anything to the patient. Therefore, memorizing and practicing how to interpret abbreviations and acronyms in healthcare is very important.

27

SUMMARIZATION

LEARNING GOAL

► After successful completion of the Summarization chapter, participants will be able to know when they are allowed to summarize and how they can advocate effectively.

LEARNING OBJECTIVES:

Using the above goals, participants should also be able to do the following upon successful completion of this chapter:

► Understand and explain when they can summarize.

► Know the role of patient advocate.

► Realize the appropriate situations for the role of Patient Advocate.

► Understand how they can overcome the systemic barriers.

► Learn how to advocate for the patient.

IMPORTANT TERMS AND WORDS

- Triggers
- Omissions
- Irrelevant
- Intercultural issues
- Systemic barrier
- Sexual orientation
- Gender identity
- Race
- Judgment

- Eligibility criteria
- Phraseology
- Intimidated
- Sexism
- Retaliation
- Exaggerated perception
- Derogatory remarks
- Derogatory side-conversations
- De-escalation strategies

Earlier this course briefly discussed summarization as a mode of interpretation. Summarization is to be avoided since it departs from the interpreter's activity of accurately and completely conveying a message from source language to target language.

Nevertheless, sometimes summarization is appropriate. Below are some situations in which you might need to use the summarization mode.

SITUATIONS THAT JUSTIFY THE SUMMARIZATION MODE

Some typical triggers for using summarization mode are when one party speaks at length and the interpreter cannot interpret simultaneously, for whatever reason, or when two or more people speak at the same time. When this happens, the interpreter should interpret the communication as completely as possible but may need to shorten or omit some ideas (*i.e.* summarize). Or depending on the situation, the interpreter can ask each party to repeat what they just stated so that it can be interpreted accurately and completely.

Summarization is generally not recommended because of the great potential for errors and omissions. Summarization should never be used as a technique for editing material that the interpreter feels is irrelevant or inappropriate. If a provider is speaking too fast, ask the provider to speak slower, instead of using summarization. If the situation requires simultaneous interpretation, perhaps another interpreter should be called.

Another situation that may be appropriate for summarization is when there is a terminologically complex third-party discussion (such as between two therapists) in front of a patient, but no one is speaking to the patient. The interpreter will then interpret simultaneously for the patient. However, if the density of the content is such that it is difficult for the interpreter to contain all the information, summarization will be in order. They may not be able to speak slowly to each other for the benefit of the patient.

THE ROLE OF PATIENT ADVOCATE

The term 'advocacy' is misunderstood. In many languages it means representation, but in English it has two meanings. One is representation, but the other is promotion. For example, if one is an advocate for communication, one will take actions to ensure that communication takes place. If one is an advocate for language access, one will alert the provider of the need for language access, such as by suggesting that a document needs to be translated for the patient instead of sight translated due to its length. If one is an advocate for client education, one will use every opportunity to educate clients (providers, patients, agencies) on the work of medical interpreters. If one is an intercultural advocate, one will work hard to alert all on the intercultural issues that actually may affect the quality of care.

However, when we speak of patient advocacy (or the patient advocate role), we are speaking of representing the best interests of the patient, usually against someone or a situation. Unlike the roles of conduit, clarifier, and cultural mediator, the role of patient advocate within an interpreting session is not a neutral role. Therefore, this role is the most invasive of all, since it means the interpreter must take the side of one of the parties, which

is contrary to the ethical goal of impartiality that every mediator needs to have.

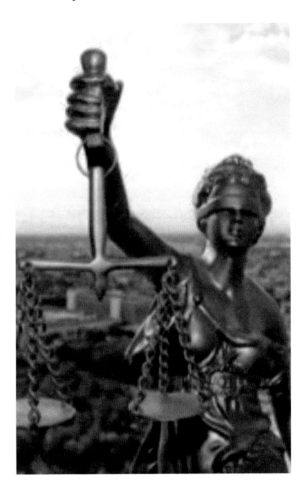

APPROPRIATE SITUATIONS FOR THE ROLE OF PATIENT ADVOCATE

First of all, in order to establish impartiality, the interpreter is supposed to avoid taking sides. However, patient advocacy is a *role* that requires taking the side of the patient. Remember from the first day of the course that modes are the *method* of interpretation, while roles are *functions* played in order to problem solve.

In all medical interpreting standards, patient advocacy is an appropriate role only where a patient's life, health, or dignity is at risk. This role can be tempting for interpreters as many enter the profession with the idea to help patients. However, interpreters work for patients and providers equally. This role has been construed as the interpreter's attempts to put the patient at the same level as the provider. The mere presence of the interpreter acts as a balancing effect relative to the power differential between the patient and the interpreter. The interpreter does not need to take any further action to ensure that the patient is well represented as that may be seen as assuming the provider doesn't have the patient's best interest in mind. This may put the provider in a defensive position. It is not needed when the patient faces a one-time inconvenience. All patients face inconveniences every day. Representing the patient is not the role of the interpreter. Representing both parties equally is.

In this course, a patient's dignity includes not only physical dignity (e.g. privacy when changing clothes) but also dignity in the face of systemic barrier as we mentioned earlier in the code of ethics and standards of practice section.

OVERCOMING SYSTEMIC BARRIERS
....

When a provider or important service rejects or otherwise discriminates against a patient because of his or her race, national origin, religion, sexual orientation, gender identity, or other similar characteristic, the interpreter has the duty of advocating for the patient. However, this does not mean that the interpreter has to take any action in front of the provider and the patient.

Interpreters should use careful judgment when evaluating whether a problem was caused by a systemic barrier. Remember that patient advocacy is needed only in certain situations.

SYSTEMIC BARRIERS are policies, practices or procedures that result in some people receiving unequal access or being excluded. Example: eligibility criteria that effectively exclude people based on a disability.

Source: http://www.accessibilitymb.ca/types-of-barriers.html

HOW TO ADVOCATE FOR THE PATIENT
....

During interpreting sessions, interpreters should always intervene incrementally whenever there is not a medical emergency. If an interpreter can resolve a systemic barrier without taking sides, the interpreter will enable the parties to resolve the issue themselves and will most likely be able to continue to interpret between the patient and the provider after the problem is resolved. This will take high-level soft skills and phraseology that avoids blaming sides. "The situation is (such and such)" is better than "I see you said... and she said...". This will be seen as blaming or judging and can quickly lead to unwanted interpersonal dynamics or even reprimand from the provider or patient.

Sometimes patient advocacy is the only way to solve a systemic barrier against the patient, such as discrimination. However, in these cases, interpreters should consider when to intervene. Interpreters can intervene before, during, or after an interpreting session. Since this is difficult to predict, it is almost never addressed before an encounter. However, it can happen. For example, an interpreter may warn the provider that the patient is known to be difficult or belligerent, or that the patient seems upset, in order to prepare the provider. If the interpreter is uncomfortable with the language or attitude of a provider towards the patient, or notices that the patient is uncomfortable or intimidated by the provider's behavior, the interpreter has several options. If the issue is becoming unbearable, one option is for the interpreter to ask the provider to step outside for a quick conversation that may help the session. Then once outside, the interpreter would begin by describing the perceived discomfort of the patient in the politest way (for example, stating "the patient's nonverbal language is signaling that the patient feels intimidated") and establishing that this may negatively affect the therapeutic rapport. The interpreter should also avoid discussing (judging) the provider's behavior, but instead should describe the perceived discomfort. The interpreter should never act as patient advocate in front of the patient, as that puts the provider in a very uncomfortable position and can negatively affect the provider-interpreter relationship. In addition, it would risk the provider later retaliating against the interpreter. If the interpreter and/or the patient are ignored, and the session continues with a discriminatory attitude against the patient, the interpreter may then decide to continue interpreting and choose to wait until after the session and solve the problem by reporting the behavior NOT to the provider, but to a supervisor or public official. Depending on the provider, the interpreter may request that the complaint be kept confidential. If the discrimination is subtle but is observed in many encounters (such as sexism towards several patients), the interpreter should report it to their supervisor or through the incident reporting mechanism of the organization, so that remedial action may take place for other patients not to suffer.

Interpreters should realize it is a huge responsibility to act as a patient advocate. Much care has to be taken to avoid retaliation and to ensure that the discrimination is not just an exaggerated perception. On the other hand, NOT advocating for the patient when necessary (if discrimination or dignity is at risk), would in fact equate to tacitly participating in the discrimination. As mentioned earlier, confronting the provider directly may cause more problems than not, but there are professionally polite ways to handle some issues, such as a provider attempt at a side-conversation with the interpret or that includes derogatory remarks against the patient. For example, if the provider says, "These patients should learn English", the interpreter may say 'Doctor, are you sure you want me to interpret this?'. This may be a polite manner to alert the doctor that you will not participate in derogatory side-conversations.

It is important to note that the patients are not the only ones who are discriminated against. On occasion a patient will discriminate against a provider or an interpreter. In this case, whoever is being discriminated against needs to use polite and professional language to handle these situations, which are similar to the skills necessary when working with difficult people. De-escalation strategies also can be very helpful. When the provider discriminates against the interpreter, it is very important for the interpreter to report this to their supervisor, with the exact language and behavior that was considered discriminatory so that the supervisor can keep track of whether this is a one-time occurrence or whether other interpreters come along with the same complaint. In the case of the latter, the supervisor will take the appropriate action.

• •

In summary, before acting as a patient advocate, always familiarize yourself with your agency's policies and protocols related to patient advocacy.

• •

NOTES

28

HOW AND WHEN TO USE SELF-CARE

LEARNING GOAL

► After successful completion of the How and When to Use Self-Care chapter, participants will be able to know how to deal with their daily stresses and apply some self-care strategies professionally.

LEARNING OBJECTIVES:

Using the above goals, participants should also be able to do the following upon successful completion of this chapter:

► Realize and explain how they can deal with daily stress and triggers.
► Learn how to retake control when feeling overwhelmed.

IMPORTANT TERMS AND WORDS

► Stress
► Personal commitment
► Linguistic skills
► Grasp of idioms and nuance
► Traumatic situations
► Anxiety,
► Avoidance,

► Irritableness
► A crime victim
► Sexual assault
► Secondary trauma
► Stress symptoms
► Rapid heartbeat
► Cognitive Behavioral Therapy (CBT)

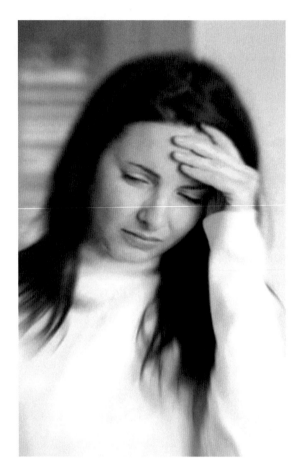

A lot of bilinguals choose to be professional medical interpreters for several reasons. Some of them come to the interpreting profession because of a personal commitment to better serve their communities and save the lives of the LEP patients. Some have worked as ad-hoc interpreters for family members or friends, so they chose this professional career to make money while using their linguistic skills to help those in great need of them. However, some of us who have been interpreters a long time feel that new interpreters may not understand that it is likely that their lives might be changed dramatically by choosing this career.

Normal stress is a part of everyday life. Any time that something unexpected or out of the routine takes place, adapting to that event can cause someone to feel stress.

Interpreting can often be very stressful, more so than people imagine. Parties expect interpreters to have great vocabulary, memory, ethics, and grasp of idioms and nuance. In addition, some interpreting fields may trigger interpreters with a history of trauma when interpreters interpret traumatic situations similar to ones they have previously experienced.

DEALING WITH STRESS AND TRIGGERS

Normal levels of stress are usually tolerable. Sometimes, however, stress is a problem. Too much stress can cause bad reactions such as nightmares, anxiety, avoidance, irritableness and depression.

For example, if a crime victim lashes out at the interpreter for misinterpreting something, that situation can be stressful and even traumatic. If the assignment runs over time, or the interpreter constantly must remind the parties to address one another, or to pause regularly, that can also be a significant source of stress.

If you interpret for victims of major trauma, even though you must actively listen to their stories, you will also need to avoid empathizing too much. When feeling overwhelmed, try to distract yourself by focusing on how each part of your body feels in that moment. Take deep breaths and ask for a break. If necessary, take several minutes to call someone and discuss something else or confide in someone and ask for their emotional support.

If an interpreting situation becomes too traumatic, you should not feel ashamed about withdrawing. It is better to take care of your own emotional health than suffer just for the sake of completing an assignment.

ADDITIONAL TRIGGERS FOR INTERPRETERS

If an interpreter has a history of experiencing domestic violence, sexual assault, or other violent crimes, the interpreter is at particular risk for developing secondary trauma.

Interpreters who have been survivors of trauma may need to manage not only their own emotional reaction of what the patient has experienced, but also the interpreter's own experience. Interpreters in these situations can experience sudden stress symptoms while interpreting, such as sweating, rapid heartbeat, or fear.

HOW TO RETAKE CONTROL WHEN FEELING OVERWHELMED

The first step to managing these reactions is to be aware of them. Then, interpreters can try to find distractions by focusing on their own bodies, taking deep breaths, and asking for a break when necessary. You should do your best to separate yourself from the story and take a break if you can. Another technique you can follow is calling someone you trust and telling them about your feelings, which can release a lot of your stress. If you have time, you can get fresh air or walk around. Washing your hands and your face is another technique that you can use to reduce some of your emotional stress.

If you cannot take a break from interpreting, try to "ground" or "center" yourself—take deep breaths and distract your negative feelings and emotions by focusing on how your toes feel, for example.

In general, the principles of mindfulness and Cognitive Behavioral Therapy (CBT) are useful starting points for additional research for interpreters who would like more guidance in these areas.

29

IDENTIFYING SECONDARY TRAUMA (VICARIOUS TRAUMA)

LEARNING GOAL

► After successful completion of the Identifying Secondary Trauma chapter, participants will be able to know how to identify and manage secondary trauma.

LEARNING OBJECTIVES:

Using the above goals, participants should also be able to do the following upon successful completion of this chapter:

► Learn how to identify the symptoms of secondary trauma.
► Define vicarious trauma.
► Learn how to remove the stigma of secondary trauma.
► Know what the patient will do if they feel secondary trauma.
► Learn valuable tips on how to deal with secondary trauma.

IMPORTANT TERMS AND WORDS

► Vicarious Trauma
► Secondary trauma
► Empathy
► Disoriented
► Neurological

► Cognitive
► Exposure
► Intrusive or distressing thoughts
► Insomnia
► Stigma

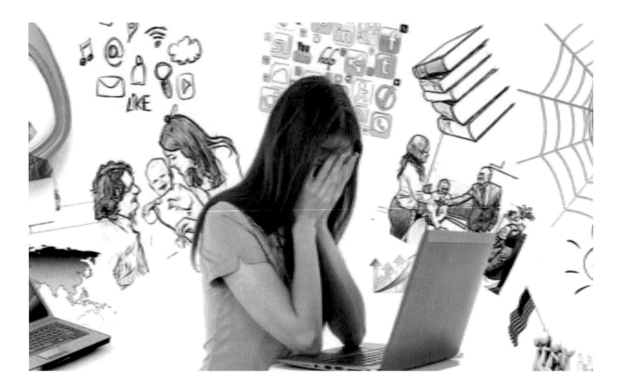

nterpreting traumatic content can be even more stressful and traumatic for interpreters than it is for many therapists, doctors, and police officers because interpreters must listen carefully, extract the meaning of a message, and deliver the message as if the event happened to them (*i.e.* in first person). Empathy is a natural emotion in interpreting because interpreters are often the voice for patients.

When interpreters are feeling especially stressed by the content of the messages they interpret, it is acceptable to switch to third person interpreting.

Before interpreters reach this point, however, they can identify and manage something called secondary trauma.

Other exceptions to using first person interpreting include if the patient is disoriented, mentally ill, or otherwise shows confusion about who is speaking.

WHAT IS VICARIOUS TRAUMA?

According to the vicarious trauma institute:

Vicarious Trauma is defined as a transformation in the helper's inner sense of identity and existence that results from utilizing controlled empathy when listening to clients' trauma-content narratives. In other words, Vicarious Trauma is what happens to your neurological (or cognitive), physical, psychological, emotional and spiritual health when you listen to traumatic stories day after day or respond to traumatic situations *while having to control your reaction.*

Resource: https://vicarioustrauma.com/ whatis.html

SECONDARY TRAUMA (VICARIOUS TRAUMA)

Vicarious trauma is also known as Secondary trauma, a buildup of exposure to the trauma others experience. Even therapists trained in secondary trauma can experience it. It means that the interpreter starts to experience some of the trauma symptoms of the people whose stories he or she hears and repeats during the interpreting session.

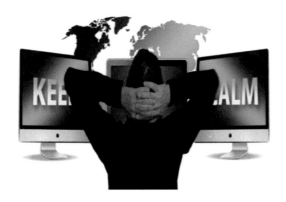

One example of secondary trauma in interpreting is when interpreters begin having nightmares about the experiences they interpret about.

Interpreters can also start to have the following secondary trauma-induced responses related to their work:

- ► Intrusive or distressing thoughts;
- ► Anxiety;
- ► Depression;
- ► Insomnia;
- ► Recurring health problems like infections;

- ► Fear for one's own safety (*eg.* fear of parking lots); or
- ► Fear for the safety of loved ones.

If you find yourself having some of these symptoms, it could mean that you are experiencing secondary trauma.

REMOVING THE STIGMA OF SECONDARY TRAUMA

Many people in the United States feel inadequate when they experience the symptoms of trauma. They may feel that they are "not tough enough" or are "being too emotional." However, secondary trauma is normal for people exposed to others' trauma. It is not a sign of weakness.

Part of overcoming secondary trauma is to remove the stigma associated with it. Interpreters can do this by no longer associating it with a personal failure and recognizing that it is often a natural consequence of working with survivors of trauma.

WHAT WILL YOU DO IF YOU FEEL SECONDARY TRAUMA?

You can follow any of the following when you feel Secondary Trauma:

- ► If you are in an interpreting session, you should ask for a break to move around and focus on something else.

- ► If you cannot take a break, you may switch to reported speech from first person (using the third-person {he, she and they} instead of the first-person {I, me, myself, and mine}).

► Realize that withdrawing and feeling secondary trauma are not weaknesses; they are recognitions of our situation.

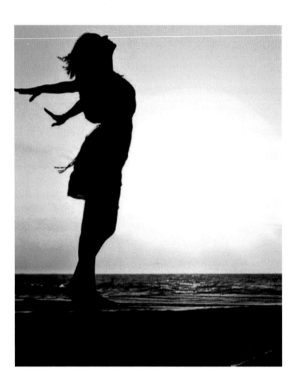

TIPS FOR DEALING WITH SECONDARY TRAUMA:

To deal with Secondary Trauma, you should follow these valuable tips to manage your feelings effectively:

► Remember stress is a part of everyday life

► Normal levels of stress are normally ok

► Sometimes you can feel too much stress

► When you feel overwhelmed, try to distract yourself or pause

► Focus on how parts of your body feel (known as "grounding")

► Take deep breaths and ask for a break

► Call someone and discuss something else

► Tell the provider about how you feel

NOTES

30

WORKING WITH TRAUMA SURVIVORS

LEARNING GOAL

► After successful completion of the Working with Trauma Survivors chapter, participants will be able to know how to work with trauma survivors during their medical interpreting encounters.

LEARNING OBJECTIVES:

Using the above goals, participants should also be able to do the following upon successful completion of this chapter:

► Learn how to work with work with trauma survivors and manage the sessions that include trauma survivors smoothly.
► Learn what the best position will be when interpreting for vulnerable groups.
► Understand and explain how they can let providers establish rapport.

IMPORTANT TERMS AND WORDS

► Trauma survivors
► Dire poverty
► Homelessness;
► Immigration detention

► Vulnerable group encounters
► Detached
► Rapport
► Second guess

TRAUMA SURVIVORS (also referred to as trauma victims) are people who have experienced **trauma**, which is the response to a deeply distressing or disturbing event that overwhelms an individual's ability to cope. (Trauma Relief | Dr. Kristin Schaefer-Schiumo, Manhasset, NY. https://www.drkristinschaeferschiumo.com/services/trauma/)

LEP trauma survivors can sometimes appear to make strange decisions. However, patients often have good reasons for their decisions. For example, an LEP person may be in one of the following situations that affects his or her decision-making:

► Dire poverty;

► Homelessness;

► Stolen documents or documents confiscated by an abuser;

► Threats from an abuser to place a victim in immigration detention;

► Threats to take the victim's children; and

► Fear of retaliation from the abuser if the victim leaves the relationship.

Unfortunately, fears of retaliation by abusers are often well-founded.

Although it may be tempting to advocate for traumatized clients with their providers, interpreters should not do so in the absence of the triggers mentioned in the "last resort" section above. Instead, the interpreter should let the provider take charge of the situation.

Providers, not interpreters, are trained to help trauma survivors process the trauma they experience. Providers such as therapists may sometimes seem to act harshly with LEP patients, but they often do so for good reasons.

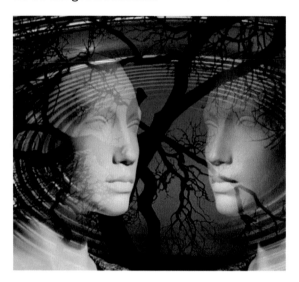

POSITIONING WHEN INTERPRETING FOR VULNERABLE GROUPS

Positioning is also unpredictable and difficult in many vulnerable group encounters because the LEP person may need additional personal space to feel safe or the LEP person may unexpectedly reach out to the interpreter when the LEP person feels strong emotions. Interpreters should conduct a pre-session whenever possible if they know they will be working with trauma survivors because the therapist or other public service provider may have special requests.

One of the most common requests from providers to interpreters when working with trauma survivors is to remain calm and detached during the interpreting session. While an interpreter's tone may reflect the emotions of the speaker, the interpreter needs to remain calm because LEP persons will detect an interpreter's distress and may become more distressed in turn.

LETTING PROVIDERS ESTABLISH RAPPORT

RAPPORT is a close relationship in which people understand each other's feelings or ideas and communicate well. Providers often try to establish good rapport with patients.

Interpreters may sometimes find that the relationship between the LEP person and the interpreter (one of at least three relationships in any interpreting session) is getting in the way of the rapport the provider is trying to establish with the patient. When this happens, interpreters should immediately signal the provider and look to the provider for cues.

Interpreters must trust the therapists and other providers they work with, even if the professionals speak in ways that puzzle or upset interpreters. Do not interfere or second-guess the provider. Be sure to follow the provider's lead.

31

RESOURCES AND ASSOCIATIONS FOR PROFESSIONAL DEVELOPMENT

LEARNING GOAL

► After successful completion of the Resources and Associations for Professional Development chapter, participants will get very helpful resources and be introduced to some non-profit associations and organizations that will help them develop their interpreting profession.

LEARNING OBJECTIVES:

Using the above goals, participants should also be able to do the following upon successful completion of this chapter:

► Gain plentiful medical interpreting resources that will help them grow professionally.
► Learn about professional interpreting organizations and associations that will help them develop their interpreting profession.
► Learn how to improve their medical terminology over time.

IMPORTANT TERMS AND WORDS

► Associations
► Professional development
► Glossaries

► A study tool
► Professional networking
► Professional forums

UNABRIDGED MONOLINGUAL DICTIONARY

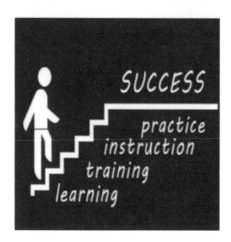

IMPROVING TERMINOLOGY OVER TIME

Every interpreter's path in interpreting is different, but many resources that interpreters use to develop themselves are the same. For example, most interpreters can improve their terminology.

Acquiring **proficiency in terminology** can take years, and interpreters must continuously strive to enhance their vocabulary. This effort requires steady work and practice. It cannot be accomplished during a single training. Instead, interpreters must prepare carefully for each assignment.

Interpreters can identify new terminology by recording the new words they encounter and then adding them to a **personal glossary** (*i.e.* a short, personal dictionary). Many modern websites, Twitter or other social media accounts, and services also offer terminology sets, or word-a-day posts.

Interpreters often create glossaries as a study tool then keep returning to them to add additional translations for words or to review what they learned from previous assignment types they need to refresh. When building a glossary, do not try to create one in a single session, week, or even month. Instead, keep slowly adding word and phrase translations to your glossary until you have a rich, personalized resource. For many interpreters, electronic documents are best because they can be edited without the need to erase or mark out old information.

ASSOCIATIONS AND ADDITIONAL RESOURCES

Second, most interpreters will benefit from **professional networking**, in addition to speaking with and learning from other interpreters. This can be done online through professional forums at ata.net, proz.com, or the forums at wordreference.com. It can also involve in-person meetings such as workshops or conferences. Some professional associations that medical interpreters should consider joining include:

► The American Translators' Association (Interpreting Division) http://www.ata-divisions.org/ID/ ;

► The National Council on Interpreting in Healthcare (NCIHC) https://www.ncihc.org/;

- The International Medical Interpreters Association https://www.imiaweb.org/; and
- The National Association of Judiciary Interpreters and Translators https://najit.org/.

Apart from compiling a glossary and professional networking, interpreters can improve by building a personal library. Some helpful resources include:

- A comprehensive or unabridged monolingual dictionary for each working language;
- ACEBO materials;
- Interpretapes; and
- Books on interpreting techniques such as Andrew Gillies' *Note-Taking for Consecutive Interpreting* and all of Holly Mickelson's works.
- The following list of resources are from IMIA Guide on Medical Interpreter Ethical Conduct. By Eva Hernandez-Iverson. (https://www.imiaweb.org/uploads/pages/376_2.pdf)

LIST SERVES

- CLAS TALK Listserv: http://www.diversityrx.org
- IMIA List serve: IMIAdiscussion@mail.imiaweb.org
- NCIHC List serve: www.ncihc.org

MEDICAL INFORMATION SITES

- Medline Plus: http://www.medlineplus.gov
- Web MD: http://www.webmd.com

ONLINE GLOSSARIES

- Language Automation, Glossaries by Language: http://www.lai.com/glossaries.html

BOOK SERVICES

- ACEBO: http://www.acebo.com
- InTrans Book Service: http://www.intransbooks.com
- John Benjamins Publishing: http://www.benjamins.com/cgi-bin/welcome.cgi

RECOMMENDED READING

- California Standards for Healthcare Interpreters: http://chiaonline.org/images/Publications/CA_standards_healthcare_interpreters.pdf
- HIPAA: http://hhs.gov/ocr/hipaa
- LEP, Language Rights: http://www.migrationinformation.org/integration/language_portal/Language_Rights_Briefing_Book.pdf

► The Commonwealth Fund: http://cmwf.org/Content/Publications/Fund-Reports/2006/Aug/Promising-Practices-for-Patient-Centered-Communication-with-Vulnerable-Populations-Examples-from-Ei.aspx

► National Library of Medicine. National Institutes of Health. Hippocratic Oath. Viewed March 13, 2009 (http://www.nlm.nih.gov/hmd/greek/greek_oath.html)

► Arocha, Izabel. 2006. Ethical Considerations. Boston University Center for Professional Education. Izabel Arocha, M.Ed.

► Office of Minority Health. 2000. National Standards on Culturally and Linguistically Appropriate Services. U.S. Department of Health and Human Services. Office of Minority Health.

► American Society for Testing and Measure Standards (ASTM). 2001. Standard Guide for Language Interpretation Services, F 2089. American Society for Testing and Measure Standards. Viewed November 10, 2009. (http://www.astm.org/Standards/F2089)

► International Medical Interpreters Association. March 2009. Ethics Survey.

► Sapir, E. 1921. Language. Harcourt, Brace & Co. New York.

► International Medical Interpreters Association. 1995. Medical Interpreting Standards of Practice. International Medical Interpreters Association and Education Development Center, Inc. Viewed March 19, 2009. (http://www.imiaweb.org/uploads/pages/102.pdf)

► U.S. Department of Health and Human Services Office for Civil Rights. Limited English Proficiency. U.S. Department of Health and Human Services. Viewed March 17, 2009 (http://www.hhs.gov/ocr/civilrights/resources/specialtopics/lep/index. html)

► Office of Minority Health. 2000. National Standards on Culturally and Linguistically Appropriate Services. U.S. Department of Health and Human Services. Office of Minority Health. Viewed November 10, 2009 (http://www.omhrc.gov/templates/browse.aspx?lvl=2&lvlID=15)

► California Healthcare Interpreters Association. 2002. California Standards for Healthcare Interpreters. California Healthcare Interpreters Association. Viewed November 10, 2009. (http://chiaonline.org/images/Publications/CA_standards_healthcare_ interpreters.pdf)

ADDITIONAL TRAINING

Lastly, interpreters should consider taking additional trainings. This is called continuing education (CE). Almost any training will help enhance an interpreter's skills, but interpreters can maximize their learning in trainings by pairing them with shadowing experiences with experienced interpreters, and by focusing on a particular field of interest in interpreting.

32

THE IMPORTANCE OF BECOMING CERTIFIED

LEARNING GOAL

► After successful completion of The Importance of Becoming Certified chapter, participants will know the importance of becoming a certified medical interpreter instead of a qualified medical interpreter.

LEARNING OBJECTIVES:

Using the above goals, participants should also be able to do the following upon successful completion of this chapter:

► Learn the main differences between certificate and certification, qualified vs certified.
► Know the two organizations (CCHI and NBCMI) that certify medical interpreters who speak certain languages.
► Know the differences between the two organizations (CCHI and NBCMI) that certify medical interpreters.
► Learn important tips on how to be certified.

IMPORTANT TERMS AND WORDS

► CCHI and NBCMI
► Certified Medical Interpreter (CMI)
► Certified Healthcare Interpreter (CHI)
► Certification
► Credentialing Excellence
► Prestigious credential
► Core Certification Healthcare Interpreter™ (CoreCHI™)

The Academy of Interpretation's Medical Interpreting Course is a foundational course that gives qualifying students either a completion or attendance certificate at the end of the course. This certificate should not be confused with **certification**, which means passing one of the two major tests administered for medical interpreters in the United States.

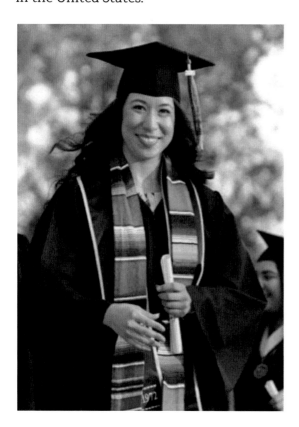

WHAT IS CERTIFICATION?

The Institute for Credentialing Excellence (formerly NOCA), established by Congress to develop standards for quality certification in the allied health fields, says,

The certification of specialized skill-sets affirms a knowledge and experience base for practitioners in a particular field, their employers, and the public at large. Certification represents a declaration of a particular individual's professional competence.

Source: https://www.ncihc.org/ certification

WHAT IS DEFINITION OF THE HEALTHCARE MEDICAL INTERPRETING CERTIFICATION?

According to The National Board of Certification for Medical Interpreters website, the healthcare medical interpreting certification is the most prestigious credential which is considered an entry-level certification for medical interpreters who meet industry-standard educational requirements and pass a written and oral examination. These exams test adequate knowledge of the medical interpreting profession, including ethics, standards of practice, role boundaries and medical terminology, among other important competencies; (Program Overview—MemberClicks (https://nbcmi. memberclicks.net/overview). The National Board of Certification for Medical Interpreters website: https://www.certifiedmedicalinterpreters.org/overview.

These tests are offered by the National Board of Certification for Medical Interpreters (NBCMI) or Certification Commission for Healthcare Interpreters (CCHI) Certified Healthcare Interpreter (CHI). We will discuss the differences between both of them shortly.

MAKING CERTIFICATION YOUR GOAL

Professional certification is an important mark of a profession, as it means there are officially accepted and recognized mechanisms to certify that an individual is competent to practice a particular profession. While national certification has been available to medical interpreters since 2009, interpreters are not required by law to be certified to interpret. However, many healthcare organizations are requiring it or listing certification as a preference. Certification allows interpreters to prove to agencies and providers that they are competent and knowledgeable in interpreting. Additionally, certification often allows interpreters to charge higher rates.

All medical interpreters should make certification an important career goal. Working towards certification and maintaining certification helps interpreters improve.

In the United States, the two major agencies that offer national certification are the **Certification Commission for Healthcare Interpreters (CCHI)** http://cchicertification.org/ and the **National Board of Certification for Medical Interpreters (NBCMI)** https://www.certifiedmedicalinterpreters.org/. While interpreters just need to get certified by one organization in order to be called a certified interpreter, some interpreters have decided to become certified by both organizations to differentiate themselves from other colleagues and gain a marketing and branding advantage.

DIFFERENCES BETWEEN THE CCHI AND NBCMI CERTIFICATION PROGRAMS

According to its website, CCHI offers two national credentials for medical interpreters: the Core Certification Healthcare Interpreter™ (CoreCHI™) and Certified Healthcare Interpreter™ (CHI™).

The CCHI written exam evaluates an interpreter's knowledge about healthcare interpreting. It is in English and has 100 questions total from the following topics: professional responsibility and interpreter ethics, managing the interpreting encounter, healthcare terminology, US healthcare systems, and cultural responsiveness. CCHI offers the CoreCHI™ credential to all interpreters who do not interpret into Arabic, Spanish, and Mandarin. To obtain the CoreCHI credential, the candidate must pass the CCHI written exam only.

The CHI Credential is offered to those that interpret into Arabic, Spanish, and Mandarin, and requires candidates to pass the written CCHI exam and also to pass the oral CCHI Exam, which evaluates an interpreter's skills in interpreting in healthcare. The oral CCHI exam includes consecutive, simultaneous, and sight translation modes. In order to receive the CHI™ credential an interpreter needs to pass both the oral and the written exams. The CCHI credentials last four (4) years.

According to the NBCMI website, NBCMI offers one credential, the Certified Medical Interpreter (CMI) credential. The NBCMI written exam tests adequate knowledge of the medical interpreting profession, including ethics, standards of practice, role boundaries and medical terminology, among other competencies. It is important to note that 75% of the exam relates to medical terminology. As of the date of publishing, the oral exam is offered in six languages: Spanish, Cantonese, Mandarin, Russian, Korean, and Vietnamese. The oral exam includes consecutive and sight translation modes. In order to receive the CMI credential an interpreter needs to pass both the oral and the written exams. The NBCMI CMI credential lasts five (5) years.

Both organizations require continuing education units (CEUs). IMIA requires 30 hours of continuing education in 5 years CCHI requires 32 hours of continuing education in 4 years. Both require certificates or other proof of completion of CEUs in order to recertify.

SOME ADVANTAGES OF CERTIFICATION

- ► More assignments
- ► Higher pay
- ► Greater variety of assignments
- ► Easier way to prove your training
- ► Preparation helps you improve

ADDITIONAL TIPS TO PREPARE FOR CERTIFICATION

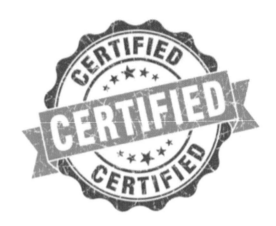

- ► Set long-term goals
Many interpreters start preparing a year or more in advance

- ► Buy preparation materials
Many authors have written preparation materials, not only Holly Mikkelson (https://www.middlebury.edu/institute/people/holly-mikkelson)

- ► Ask someone to hold you accountable
You are more likely to achieve your goals when you are responsible to someone

- ► Don't be afraid to ask for help!

Many of your colleagues are struggling or have struggled with the same problems

NOTES

33

LIABILITY INSURANCE

LEARNING GOAL

► After successful completion of the Liability Insurance chapter, participants will know how to get a liability insurance as professional interpreters.

LEARNING OBJECTIVES:

Using the above goals, participants should also be able to do the following upon successful completion of this chapter:

► Learn and explain the interpreters' liability insurance that can cover them in case of omissions or errors.

IMPORTANT TERMS AND WORDS

► Liability coverage for errors and omissions

► Claims process

ew interpreters immediately think of being sued when starting their careers (and statistics show that few interpreters are in fact sued). Nevertheless, many interpreters, agencies, and parties prefer to have or work with interpreters who have liability coverage for errors and omissions.

When choosing liability insurance coverage, be sure to ask about exclusions, deductibles, and the claims process. Some insurance companies will take an active role in litigation if you are ever sued; others will not.

Liability insurance is more broadly a part of how you want to present yourself to agencies, freelance clients, and other interpreters: does your brand carry a guarantee of accuracy, and can you back up that guarantee with insurance?

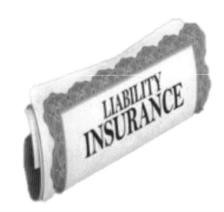

NOTES

34

SELF-MONITORING AND SELF-ASSESSMENT

LEARNING GOAL

► After successful completion of the Self-Monitoring and Self-Assessment chapter, participants will know how to perform self-monitoring and self-assessment on a daily or weekly basis to help them grow professionally.

LEARNING OBJECTIVES:

Using the above goals, participants should also be able to do the following upon successful completion of this chapter:

► Learn and explain all the self-monitoring and self-assessment techniques that they can perform on daily or weekly basis to increase self-esteem and help them grow professionally.

► Learn how to make their goals SMART.

IMPORTANT TERMS AND WORDS

► Self-monitoring and self-assessment

► Shadowing

► Measurable, Attainable, timely

► Acronym

Professional athletes exercise daily, and serious language-learners speak and learn daily because both groups know that they need to always be improving to reach their goals. Just like a professional athlete or serious language-learner, you can set goals and improve regularly.

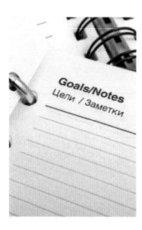

First, a goal that is not written is merely a dream. Take the time to sit down and write out your interpreting goals. Some of those goals may include learning field-specific vocabulary (e.g. medical terminology), becoming certified, interpreting for a certain number of hours per week through shadowing other interpreters, practicing note-taking outside of interpreting sessions, or other means that will help you achieve all your professional goals.

When setting goals, always make your goals SMART:

SPECIFIC,
MEASURABLE,
ATTAINABLE,
RELEVANT,
TIMELY.

Specific goals are expressed in a way that makes it easy to determine what you are aiming for. "I want to get better at note-taking" is not a specific goal, but "I will practice note-taking by listening to recorded speeches" is specific. Next, make sure your goal is measurable. In the previous example, you might add a time element such as "for 15 minutes per day." Depending on your goal, you may instead opt to measure an outcome such as "learn five new medical terms per day."

Third, attainable goals are those that push you to improve without making you feel overwhelmed. Be excited about your goals, but do not be too hard on yourself when you fall short. No one meets 100 percent of their goals. Part of self-assessment is accepting yourself for who and where you are on your professional path and adjusting your goals to be more attainable as you learn.

The last two letters of the "SMART" acronym stand for relevant and timely. Relevant goals focus on your needs as an interpreter. If you already have great note-taking skills, for example, you will not need to set goals to learn about note-taking (although it may still be appropriate to practice). Timely goals, on the other hand, are those with an appropriate deadline. When setting a timely goal, you might include language such as "for the next three months" or "by June 1." Lastly, involve a friend or close colleague in your goals and report to them when appropriate. You are more likely to follow through on your goals when you are accountable to someone else.

Goal setting is a skill that requires practice and patience just like exercising, language-learning, and interpreting. As you improve your goal-setting skills, your interpreting skills will also benefit.

REFERENCES CITED

Angelelli, C. (2004). Medical Interpreting and Cross-cultural Communication. Cambridge: Cambridge University Press. doi:10.1017/CBO9780511486616

Angelelli, C.V. (2004b). Revisiting the interpreters' roles: A study of conference, court, and medical interpreters in Canada, Mexico, and the United States. Amsterdam: Benjamin.

California Healthcare Interpreters Association, C., 2002. California Standards for Healthcare Interpreters. Chiaonline.org. From, http://www.chiaonline.org/Resources/Documents/CHIA%20Standards/standards_chia.pdf

Chavez, J. M. (1993, February). Breaking through the language barrier. Urban Medicine.

CHIA Standards & Certification Committee, California Healthcare Interpreters Association. California Standards for Healthcare Interpreters: Ethical Principles, Protocols, and Guidance on Roles & Intervention. 2002. Los Angles, CA: CHIA.

Dean, R. K., & Pollard, R. Q. (2005). Consumers and service effectiveness in interpreting work: A practice profession perspective. In M. Marschark, R. Peterson, & E. A. Winston (Eds.), Sign Language Interpreting and Interpreter Education (pp. 259- 282). Retrieved from https://intrprgithub.io/library/dean-pollard-practiceprofessions.pdf

Gish, S. (1987). I understood all the words, but I missed the point: A goal-to-detail/detail-to-goal strategy for text analysis. In M. McIntire (Ed.), New dimensions in interpreter education—curriculum and instruction, Silver Spring, MD: RID Publications.

Health, C. What is Telemedicine?: Telemedicine System. From https://chironhealth.com/telemedicine/what-is-telemedicine/

Holt Barrett, K. (2005). Guidelines for conducting successful cross-cultural evaluations. In K. Holt Barrett, & W. H. George (Eds.), Race culture, psychology and law. New York: Sage.

Hsieh, E. (2006a). Conflicts in how interpreters manage their roles in provider-patient interactions. Social Science & Medicine , 62, 721-730.

Hsieh, E. (2006b). Understanding medical interpreters: Reconceptualizing bilingual health communication. Health Communication, 20, 177-186.

Humphrey, J. H., & Alcorn, B. J. (1995). So you want to be an interpreter?: An introduction to sign language interpreting. Amarillo, TX: H & H Publishers.

Jackson-Carroll, L. M., Graham, E., & Jackson, J. C. (1996). Beyond medical interpretation: The role of interpreters cultural mediators. In *Building bridges between ethnic communities and health institutions.* https://www.hslib. washington.edu/clinical/ethnomed/ ICM/.

Kaufert, J. M., & Koolage, W. W. (1984). Role conflict among culture brokers: The experience of Native Canadian medical interpreters. *Social Science and Medicine, 18*(3), 283-286.

Kaufert, J. M., O'Neil, J. D., & Koolage, W. W. (1985). Culture brokerage and advocacy in urban hospitals: The impact of Native language interpreters. *Sante Culture Health, 2*(3), 3-9.

Kelly. (2000). Cultural parameters for interpreters in the courtroom. The Critical Link 2: Interpreters in the Community, Selected papers from the Second International Conference on Interpreting in legal, health and social service settings, 131-148. Philadelphia, PA: John Benjamins.

Leanza, Y. (2005). Le rapport à l'autre culturel en milieu médical. L'exemple de consultations pédiatriques de prévention pour des familles migrantes. Bulletin de l'Association pour la Recherche InterCulturelle 41, 8-27.

Metzger. M. (1995). The paradox of neutrality: A comparison of interpreters' goals with the realities of interactive discourse. Phd dissertation, Georgetown University.

Metzger, M. (1999) Sign language interpreting: Deconstructing the myth of neutrality. Washington, DC: Gallaudet University Press.

Metzger, M., E. Fleetwood & S. Collins. (2004). "Discourse genre and linguistic mode: Interpreter influences in visual and tactile interaction". Sign Language Studies. 4(2), 118-137

Orellana, M., & Dana Brems, D. (2017). Limitations of Ad Hoc Interpreters on Patient Understanding and Compliance in Diabetic Foot Care. From https://www.academia.edu/27263750/ Limitations_of_Ad_Hoc_Interpreters_ on_Patient_Understanding_and_ Compliance_in_Diabetic_Foot_ Care?email_work_card=thumbnail

Pöchhacker, F. (n.d.). Introducing Interpreting Studies (2, revised ed.). Routledge, 2016.

Pöchhacker, Franz and Miriam Shlesinger (eds) (2002). The Interpreting Studies Reader. London and New York : Routledge. 436 pages. ISBN 0- 415-22477-2 (hbk). Isbn 0-415-22478-0 (pbk)

Putsch, R. W. (1990). Language in cross-cultural care. In H. K. Walker, W. D. Hall, & J. W. Hurst (Eds.), *Clinical methods* (3rd ed., pp. 1060-1065). Boston: Butterworths.

Putsch, R. W. & Joyce, M. (1990). Dealing with patients from other cultures. In H. K. Walker, W. D. Hall, & J. W. Hurst (Eds.), *Clinical methods* (3rd ed., pp. 1050-1065). Boston: Butterworth.

Quirk, Randolph & Greenbaum, Sidney. (1998) A University Grammar Of English. London: Longman Group Ltd.

Ressler, C. (1999). "Direct interpretation and an intermediary interpretation". Journal of Interpretation.

Raval, H. (2005). Being heard and understood in the context of seeking asylum and refuge: Communicating with the help of bilingual co-workers. Clinical Child Psychology and Psychiatry, 10, 197–216.

Raval, H., & Smith, J. (2003). Therapists' experiences of working with language interpreters. International Journal of Mental Health, 32, 6–31. Razban, M. (2003). An interpreter's perspective. In R.

Roat, C. E., et. al. (1999). Bridging the Gap: A Basic Training for Medical Interpreters: Interpreter's Handbook (3rd (1st Edition–1996) ed.). Seattle, Washington: Cross Cultural Health Care Program of Pacific Medical Clinics.

Roy, C. (2000). Interpreting as a discourse process. Oxford: Oxford University Press

Sasso, A. (2000). Interpreter services in health care: A call for provincial standards and services. Vancouver: Affiliation of multicultural services agencies and societies of British Columbia.

Seleskovitch, D. (1975/2002). "Language and memory: A study of note taking in consecutive interpreting". F. Pöchhacker & M. Shlesinger (eds). The Interpreting Studies Reader. London/New York: Routledge.

Solis, J., Marks, G., Garcia, M. & Shelton, D. (1990). Acculturation, access to care, and use of preventive services by Hispanics: Findings from HHANES 1982-84. American Journal of Public Health 80 Suppl, 11-19

Souza, I. E. (2016) Intercultural Mediation in Healthcare, Xlibris Publishing, Bloomington, Indiana.

Takeda, Kayoko. (2009). The Interpreter, the Monitor and the Language Arbiter. Meta. 54. 191-200. 10.7202/037675ar.

The Joint Commission. (2010): Advancing Effective Communication, Cultural Competence, and Patient- and Family-Centered Care: A Roadmap for Hospitals. Oakbrook Terrace, IL: The Joint Commission.

Tribe, & H. Raval (Eds.), Undertaking mental health work using interpreters. London: Routledge

Wadensjö, C. (1998). Interpreting as interaction. London/New York: Longman.

Watson, J. (1987). "Interpreter burnout". Journal of Interpretation.

Woloshin, S., Schwartz, L. M., Katz, S. J. & Welch, H. G. (1997). Is language a barrier to the use of preventive services? Journal of General Internal Medicine 12 (8), 472-477.